Marie

"How are you feeling? What colors do you like? How would you want to decorate the living room?"

These were questions that I was not able to answer. I think that I used to be able to answer them, maybe as a kid, but I can't remember. I don't know who I am, how I am or what I like because I don't exist anymore. And that might be a good thing, because I couldn't bear living with me any longer —ever since I grew up. This was when I took refuge in the gray spot – a relationship with my partner, later husband, where we were both liberated from the painful existence as individuals and merged into one - one gray spot.

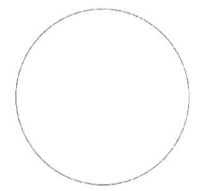 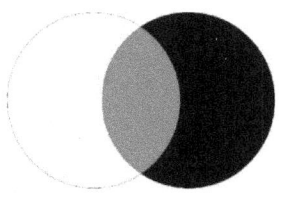 

ESCAPING THE GRAY SPOT

A COLORFUL JOURNEY OF SELF-DISCOVERY

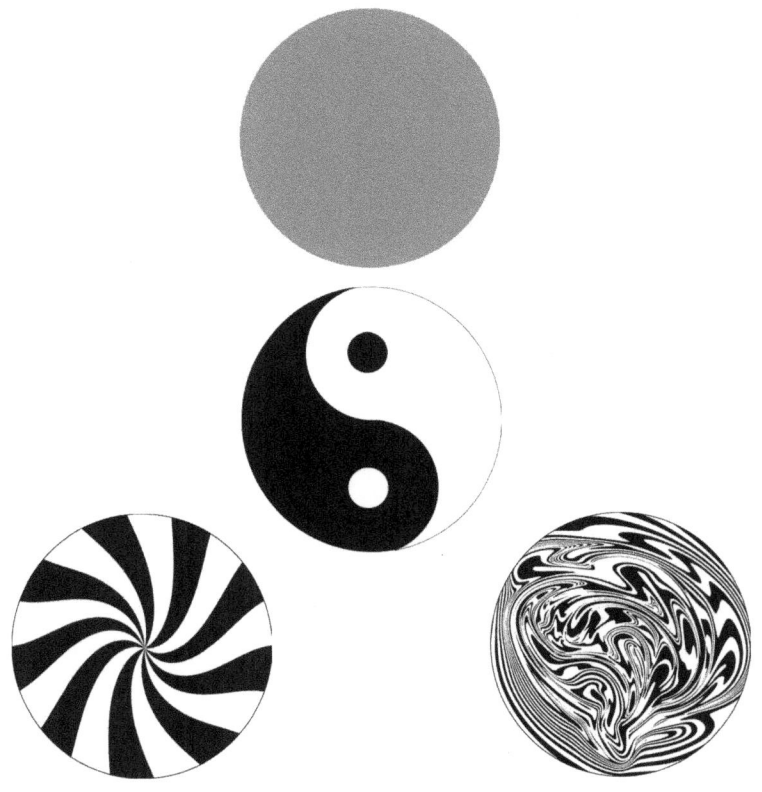

GIL ROCHAT

Table Of Contents

1   How to use this book..2

2   Acknowledgment...4

3   Prologue 6

4   Introduction..10

5   Happiness – General concepts 14

    5.1   Looking for happiness 15

    5.2   Embarking on the Journey to Inner Harmony: Understanding the Mechanisms of Happiness...25

6   Who am I and who do I want to be? 30

    6.1   The Journey of Self-Integration: Navigating the Depths of Human Nature - The "selfishness" model...31

    6.2   Understanding Your Roots 38

    6.3   Unveiling Personal Values 65

    6.4   Creating Your Guiding Principles..78

    6.5   Dream Exploration: Unveiling Your Deepest Desires 95

    6.6   Set practical objectives and related actions.........................108

7   "The Gray Spot" model...122

    7.1   Foundations of Happiness: Understanding and Cultivating Supporting Pillars 128

    7.2   "The Gray Spot": Harmonizing individuality with unity in relationships 137

    7.3   Implementing "The Gray Spot" strategies: A roadmap to personal evolution 146

8   Epilogue – Beyond "The Gray Spot" – Jump in!..............................156

9   References..162

10   Appendices 170

1 How to use this book

About the book

Entitled *'Escaping the Gray Spot – A colorful journey of self-discovery,'* this book serves as a voyage into self-awareness, delving into the intricacies of human nature from egocentrism to interconnectedness and the development of relationships. Structured to lead readers on a multifaceted expedition of self-discovery, personal development, and satisfaction. It is then segmented into various sections, each tackling distinct facets of happiness, self-awareness, personal ethics, values, and life principles, supported by personal narratives and inspiring stories from worldwide personalities.

How to navigate the content?

- Commence by reading the Prologue (Section 3) and the introduction (Section 4) to grasp the author's viewpoint and the book's intent.
- Delve into the segments on happiness (Section 5) and self-awareness (Section 6) to garner insights into the elements fostering happiness and the journey of self-understanding. Reflect upon the portions concerning personal values and principles to recognize and prioritize your fundamental values and formulate a set of principles or a personal code to steer your decision-making and conduct.
- Develop your own interpretation of "The Gray Spot" model by identifying the pillars supporting your life and determining how you want your personal journey to unfold (Section 7).
- Employ the book as a resource and guide, revisiting segments as necessary to deepen comprehension and apply the concepts to your own life.
- Participate in the suggested exercises and activities to implement the concepts and reap their rewards firsthand.

Interconnectedness of sections

- The sections are interlinked, progressively building upon one another to furnish a comprehensive comprehension of the concepts and principles elucidated in the book.
- Nevertheless, each section retains autonomy, addressing specific themes and furnishing insights and practical guidance individually.

Additional tips and recommendations for utilizing this book

- Allocate ample time to absorb and contemplate the content. This book is crafted to steer you on a journey of self-discovery, thus dedicating time to fully engage with the material is paramount.
- Embrace the opportunity to revisit segments or concepts that strike a chord with you. This book is intended to serve as a resource and guide, so feel empowered to return to sections that resonate or prove particularly enlightening.
- Contemplate discussing the concepts and ideas presented in the book with others. Sharing your musings and insights with peers, family, or a support network can deepen comprehension and furnish alternative viewpoints.
- Implement the concepts and principles outlined in the book into your own life. Participate in the suggested exercises and activities to translate the concepts into action and experience their benefits firsthand.
- Keep in mind that self-discovery is a journey, not a destination. Extend patience and kindness to yourself as you explore and evolve.

2 Acknowledgment

Writing this book has been a transformative journey, one that I could never have completed without the support, wisdom, and love of many incredible people.

To Catherine, Elise, Ivonne, Jeremy, Jean-Louis, Rebecca, Carla, Hugo, Reem and all those who took the time to read the early drafts of this book, your feedback, insights, and encouragement were invaluable. Thank you for helping me refine my ideas and for believing in the message I hoped to convey.

To Marie who generously shared her stories and anecdotes, your courage and authenticity inspired the heart of this book. Your experiences not only enriched the pages but also gave it life.

To my family and friends, who stood by me every step of the way—your unwavering support, patience, and love sustained me through this journey. A special thank you to my amazing daughter Tali, whose talent and creativity brought this book to life in a whole new way. Your illustrations added depth and vibrancy, making the concept of "The Gray Spot" not only meaningful but also visually engaging. I am so proud of you and grateful for the gift you have shared with this project.

Finally, to you, the reader: this book is a testament to the belief that growth is always possible and that each of us has the power to create meaningful change in our lives. Thank you for letting me be a part of your journey.

With gratitude,

Gil

3   Prologue

"Your time is limited, don't waste it living someone else's life."

Steve Jobs - Co-founder of Apple Inc.

"Happiness is not a goal; it is a by-product of a life well-lived."

Eleanor Roosevelt – Former US First Lady, Activist

Getting lost in this relationship was comforting. It shielded me from pain, fear, and the guilt of being me. His black and my white blended into our cozy, safe gray. For years, we were a happy gray spot, a perfect couple. But as we existed only as a couple and not as individuals, over time dependence took hold of us.

We became less mobile, less free, and more depressed. Every decision felt like a negotiation, tied to the balance of our shared existence. It felt suffocating. Then, from deep within the gray spot, a part of me started fighting to survive. That was the start of my life crisis. It was tough but it was necessary to heal.

Throughout this book, I am sharing parts of Marie's narrative. Her telling me this story, coupled with my own experience, was the start of writing it. My aspiration is that this can help others in their pursuit of happiness, whether by aiding them through crises or steering them away from getting lost in the gray spot in the first place—that's my hope.

4   Introduction

"Our lives begin to end the day we become silent about things that matter."

Martin Luther King Jr. - American Baptist minister and leader in the civil rights movement

"The privilege of a lifetime is to become who you truly are."

Carl Jung - Swiss psychiatrist and psychoanalyst.

In the pursuit of personal growth and navigating the ever-evolving landscape of our lives, there exists a fundamental truth: understanding, nurturing, and embracing our personal identity is paramount. It is the compass that guides us towards becoming our best selves, fulfilling our aspirations, and carving out our niche in a world that is in a perpetual state of flux. Without this clarity of self, we risk succumbing to a colorless existence, where the vibrancy of life fades into a monotonous, blurred gray spot.

As President Abraham Lincoln once famously remarked, "The best way to predict the future is to create it." His words resonate with the essence of proactive self-determination, urging us to seize control of our destinies with unwavering conviction. Lincoln's own legacy epitomizes the power of resilience, perseverance, and unwavering commitment to one's dreams, even in the face of seemingly insurmountable challenges.

But how do we ensure that the actions we take today pave the path towards the future we envision? This question lies at the heart of our quest for self-discovery and personal fulfilment. It beckons us to embark on a journey of introspection, guided by both managerial pragmatism and psychological insight developed and popularized by the management guru Peter Drucker and of founder of psychoanalysis, Sigmund Freud.

"The Management Insight "

Peter Drucker's management philosophy emphasizes strategic planning and proactive decision-making to shape one's future. Just as organizations define objectives and strategies to achieve success, individuals can articulate a compelling vision grounded in their strengths and values. Drucker's maxim, consistently retaken from Lincoln's, "The best way to predict the future is to create it," underscores the proactive agency individuals possess in molding their destinies.

The managerial approach implores us to articulate a compelling vision of our future selves grounded in our unique strengths and core values. By delineating our aspirations, defining what success truly means to us and aligning actions with a well-defined vision, we unlock a roadmap to personal achievement and fulfilment. This prompts soul-searching inquiries: What does success signify in the context of my life? What values underpin my existence? What innate strengths can I leverage to realize my ambitions? Crafting a vision that resonates with our essence ignites a sense of purpose and direction, propelling us towards our desired destination.

"The Psychologist Insight "

Sigmund Freud's psychoanalytic theory delves into the subconscious influences that shape human behavior and motivations. By exploring childhood experiences and unconscious drives, individuals gain insights into the internal forces that govern their lives. Freud's approach highlights the interconnectedness of past experiences with present aspirations, emphasizing the importance of reconciling past traumas with future goals.

This psychological perspective explores the intricacies of our past experiences, probing the depths of our subconscious to illuminate the path forward, paving the way for personal growth and fulfilment. Drawing from Freudian principles, this approach invites introspection into our formative years and the imprint they have left on our psyche. By unravelling the threads of our past, we glean invaluable insights into our emotional landscape, internal conflicts and cultivate a deeper understanding of ourselves. However, it also leaves us grappling with unanswered questions: How do our past experiences shape our future aspirations? How can we reconcile our past traumas with our present desires? How do we harness the wisdom gleaned from our past to cultivate a more fulfilling future?

These insights offer complementary perspectives, blending strategic foresight with emotional introspection to empower individuals in their journey towards self-discovery and personal development. It is a multifaceted quest to unearth the essence of our being, to align our actions with our authentic selves, and to forge a future that resonates with our deepest aspirations. As we navigate this odyssey, let us heed the wisdom of Drucker and Freud, seizing the reins of our destiny and sculpting a future that is uniquely our own. For in the tapestry of our lives, it is our personal identity that imbues each thread with meaning and purpose, illuminating the path towards a life well-lived.

5 Happiness – General concepts

"The happiness of your life depends upon the quality of your thoughts."

Marcus Aurelius - Roman Emperor, Stoic philosopher

"The key to being happy is knowing you have the power to choose what to accept and what to let go."

Dodinsky - Author and illustrator

5.1   Looking for happiness

"Happiness is not in the mere possession of money; it lies in the joy of achievement, in the thrill of creative effort."

Franklin D. Roosevelt - Former President of the United States

"The satisfaction of these needs is not merely a matter of survival; it forms the bedrock upon which our happiness is built"

Abraham Maslow - psychologist

Objectives of the section

Explore the multifaceted concept of happiness, delving into various aspects such as its psychological underpinnings, the balance between selfishness and selflessness, and cultural perspectives on purposeful living and well-being.

Key topics

UNDERSTAND HUMAN NEEDS - Explore how fundamental human needs contribute to happiness, as outlined in Maslow's hierarchy of needs.

BALANCE SELF AND OTHERS - Investigate how balancing personal needs with concern for others influences happiness.

CULTURAL APPROACH TO HAPPINESS - Examine how different cultures pursue happiness and purposeful living.

The search for happiness is something we have all been on at some point, right? It is like this big puzzle we have been trying to solve forever, to unravel its mysteries. Different areas like sports, philosophy, psychology, religion, and sociology have all taken a crack at figuring out what makes us happy, intertwining the perception of happiness with both physical and mental realms.

Within this intricate tapestry lie myriad factors and catalysts, crafting a complex web that shapes individuals' happiness. At its core lie values, principles, and emotions that resonate deeply within us.

Consider, for instance:

- *Health and Well-being* - Physical health, mental well-being, and self-care practices contribute significantly to overall happiness.
- *Financial Stability* - While money does not guarantee happiness, having enough resources to meet basic needs and pursue interests without excessive stress can positively impact well-being.
- *Positive Relationships* - Meaningful connections with friends, family, and community members foster feelings of belonging and support.
- *Positive Emotions* - Engaging in activities that bring joy, laughter, and excitement can boost overall happiness levels.
- *Personal Growth* - Continuous learning, self-improvement, and pursuing passions contribute to a sense of fulfilment and happiness.
- *Sense of Purpose* - Having clear goals, aspirations, and a sense of direction in life provides fulfilment and satisfaction.
- *Gratitude and Mindfulness* - Cultivating gratitude for what one has and practicing mindfulness to stay present in the moment can enhance feelings of contentment.

These elements, among others, may vary in significance for each individual, yet collectively, they play an instrumental role in shaping our overall happiness and satisfaction with life. It is incumbent upon each of us to introspect, understanding the nuanced interplay of these factors in our own lives. Only through this introspection can we strive for balance, thereby fostering a life rich in fulfilment and satisfaction.

5.1.1 From Survival to Self-Actualization: Unveiling the Layers of Human Fulfilment

In his seminal work, "A Theory of Human Motivation," penned in 1943 and published in the esteemed journal Psychological Review, Abraham Maslow laid the groundwork for what has become celebrated as Maslow's hierarchy of needs. This framework encapsulates a profound truth: that individuals must first address their fundamental needs – physiological, safety, love, and esteem – before ascending towards the pinnacle of self-actualization (Figure 1).

Figure 1- Maslow pyramid of individual psychological needs.

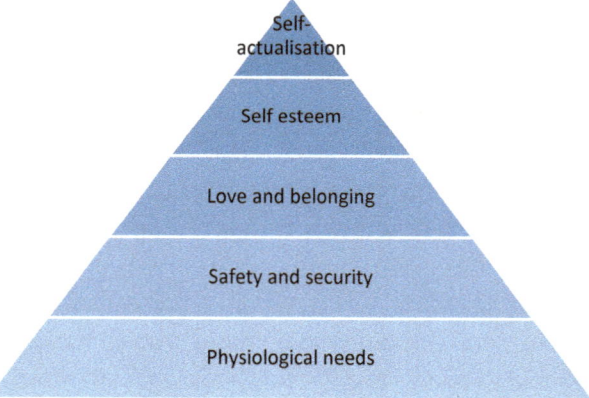

The satisfaction of these needs is not merely a matter of survival; it forms the bedrock upon which our happiness is built. Economic stability and security offer not just material comfort but a shield against the storms of stress and anxiety. And yet, it is the journey towards spiritual fulfilment, towards realizing our highest potential, that truly illuminates the path to lasting happiness.

Consider the layers of our psychological needs, from the primal requirements of sustenance and shelter to the loftier aspirations of self-realization. Each level speaks to our deepest yearnings and desires. Some insights into the specific levels of psychological needs, ranging from basic physiological requirements to higher-order aspirations related to self-actualization, are listed here.

At the base lie our *physiological needs* – the sustenance, water, shelter, sleep, and clothing essential for our physical well-being. Without these, our journey towards happiness falters before it begins.

Above this foundation, we seek *safety and security* – in our homes, our finances, our health, and our employment. These pillars fortify our existence, granting us the peace of mind necessary to pursue higher aspirations.

Love and belonging form the next stratum, weaving a tapestry of familial bonds, friendships, social connections, and community involvement. In the warmth of these relationships, we find solace and support, anchoring us amidst life's tumult.

Ascending further, we encounter the realm of *self-esteem* – where self-respect, recognition, achievement, independence, and competence reign supreme. Here, we cultivate a sense of worth and purpose, bolstering our confidence as we navigate the world.

And finally, at the summit awaits *self-actualization* – the pursuit of personal growth, creativity, knowledge, autonomy, and the fulfilment of our potential. It is here that we transcend mere existence, stepping into the fullness of our being.

Yet, the journey towards happiness is not without its complexities and is far from being linear. It is shaped not only by our values and principles but also by internal and external forces.

Internally, our values, self-awareness, emotional state, and prioritization skills guide our choices, helping us discern between genuine needs and mere desires.

Externally, we are buffeted by peer pressure, cultural norms, and economic conditions, each exerting its influence on our perception of what we require for happiness.

All these aspects contribute to personal happiness. Their impact varies from person to person based on individual values, beliefs, and priorities but also depends on personal life experiences and where we stand within our development journey, on our environment, and on our social connections. Understanding this intricate interplay is essential, for it empowers us to make decisions aligned with our true needs and long-term well-being. As we embark on our journey towards a vibrant, colorful, and fulfilling life, let us remember that true happiness arises from finding the right balance among all these elements.

5.1.2 Dance of Selfishness and Selflessness: Navigating Paths to Happiness

The interplay between selfishness and selflessness profoundly shapes our behaviors in the pursuit of personal needs and happiness.

Selfishness, characterized by a singular focus on one's own desires and needs, disregards the well-being of others. It embodies a pursuit of personal gain, often at the expense of empathy or ethical consideration. Such self-serving actions may yield fleeting gratification or success but risk fracturing social bonds and corroding meaningful relationships. When individuals prioritize their own interests without regard for the impact on others, it can foster an environment of isolation and disconnection, hindering the cultivation of deep, meaningful connections.

Conversely, selflessness embodies a noble commitment to others, prioritizing their well-being above our own. It emanates from compassion, empathy and altruism, fostering genuine connections and a shared sense of purpose. Acts of selflessness not only enrich the lives of others but also cultivate a profound sense of fulfilment within ourselves. By extending empathy and support to others, individuals create a network of reciprocal care and trust, strengthening social bonds and fostering a sense of belonging and interconnectedness.

Navigating the balance between selfishness and selflessness is paramount, reverberating through Maslow's hierarchy of needs and shaping our individual journeys toward happiness. While selfishness may momentarily satisfy basic needs and ambitions, its unchecked dominance threatens our psychological well-being and societal cohesion. Conversely, a harmonious blend of self-interest and concern for others fosters holistic well-being, propelling us toward a more meaningful existence. Striking this balance requires introspection and empathy, as individuals seek to understand their own needs while also considering the impact of their actions on others.

In summary, selfishness and selflessness intersect with Maslow's hierarchy, influencing the fulfilment of needs and, consequently, individual happiness. By cultivating a mindset of compassion and empathy, individuals can navigate this delicate balance, fostering deeper connections and a greater sense of fulfilment in both themselves and others.

5.1.3 The Happiness Mosaic: Cultural Perspectives on Purposeful Living

Throughout history, humans have sought to exert control over their lives, often through the creation of simplified models to understand and manage various aspects of existence. Happiness, a universal pursuit, is no exception to this human endeavor. Following the adage "What gets measured gets done, managed, prioritized," often attributed (most probably wrongly) to management guru Peter Drucker, the quest to find a formula for happiness persists.

In recent decades, this quest has taken concrete form, with several key drivers of happiness identified and confirmed through initiatives like the annual "World Happiness Report" published since 2002. Countries are ranked based on self-assessed life evaluations, drawing from the Gallup World Poll and analyzing six key variables:

- Income (GDP per capita)
- Physical and mental health, supported by healthy life expectancy
- Human relationships and social support, including having someone to count on in times of trouble
- Freedom to make key life decisions, encompassing respect for human rights and diversity
- Generosity and selflessness of the population
- Perceptions of internal and external corruption levels and Government Fairness

In recent years, northern European countries consistently dominate the top of these happiness rankings, reflecting robust social support systems and high standards of living.

Based on the World Happiness Report, the top 10 happiest countries in 2024 are:

1. Finland
2. Denmark
3. Iceland
4. Sweden
5. Israel

6. Netherlands
7. Norway`
8. Luxembourg
9. Switzerland
10. Australia

While these rankings offer valuable insights into the overall happiness levels of populations, they fail to account for individual specificities. Each person's perception of happiness is influenced by unique circumstances and reference points. While the World Happiness Report establishes a baseline for citizens of each country, individuals inevitably compare their personal happiness against this standard, leading to a relative interpretation of their own well-being. Therefore, it is crucial for each individual to pursue their own path to happiness, irrespective of geographical location.

Various cultures and philosophies offer diverse approaches to leading a purposeful life (refer to Appendix 1 for specific examples from various nations). Some emphasize spiritual practices and mindfulness, while others focus on personal achievements, strong social connections, nurturing relationships, or contributing to social causes or environmental sustainability, aligning their purpose with broader societal goals or the greater good.

In general, eastern philosophies like Buddhism emphasize mindfulness, meditation, and compassion, while Western societies often prioritize individual achievement and personal development.

Nations around the world implement specific policies and embrace cultural values that contribute to their residents' overall happiness. Nordic countries, for instance, prioritize social support and work-life balance, exemplified by concepts such as Finland's "Sisu," Denmark's "Hygge," and Sweden's "Lagom." Similarly, European nations like Switzerland, Italy, Netherlands, Ireland, and Greece each embody unique cultural values that foster happiness and well-being.

Across Asia, Africa, and the Americas, cultural concepts such as Japan's "Ikigai," India's "Dharma," and Ghana's "Sankofa" offer pathways to purposeful living. Whether it is embracing interconnectedness, seeking balance and harmony, or fostering community collaboration, these concepts reflect humanity's diverse approaches to finding meaning and fulfilment in life.

In conclusion, while the pursuit of happiness may be universal, the paths to achieving it are manifold, shaped by cultural traditions, societal values, and individual aspirations. By embracing the richness of these diverse perspectives, individuals and societies can cultivate a deeper understanding of happiness and lead more purposeful lives.

5.1.4   Bhutan's Path to Happiness: A Paradigm of Well-being

Though absent from the mainstream acknowledgment of the World Happiness Report, Bhutan stands out as a beacon of unconventional wisdom in the pursuit of well-being. It is not merely an interesting case; it is profoundly inspiring, embodying a fusion of health and happiness that demands attention.

At the heart of Bhutan's ethos lies its groundbreaking Gross National Happiness framework. This holistic approach evaluates happiness across nine interwoven domains, ranging from the spiritual and physical to the social and psychological. By recognizing the intrinsic value of cultural diversity, Bhutan's framework serves as a testament to the nation's commitment to inclusive well-being.

In the face of adversity, such as the COVID crisis between 2019 and 2023, Bhutan's model showcases its resilience. The framework galvanizes collective action, uniting the population to mitigate the impact of challenges. Moreover, it extends beyond rhetoric, influencing governmental metrics of success and demonstrating a profound alignment of values and policy.

The nine constituents of Gross National Happiness—psychological well-being, health, time use and balance, education, cultural diversity and resilience, good governance, community vitality, ecological diversity and resilience, and living standards—form the foundation of a society oriented towards human flourishing.

Each domain is further reinforced by specific indicators, empowering Bhutan to identify both pockets of contentment and areas in need of improvement. This strategic approach enables the nation to nurture well-being at its core, addressing fundamental human needs with precision and empathy.

Bhutan's journey serves as a poignant reminder that true progress transcends economic metrics. It is a testament to the enduring power of values, principles, and collective action in fostering a society where happiness is not just an aspiration but a shared reality.

5.2 Embarking on the Journey to Inner Harmony: Understanding the Mechanisms of Happiness

---

"Our emotions are a fine tissue woven from the threads of physiology, cognition, and environment."

Dr. Emily Johnson, Psychologist and Author of "The Science of Happiness"

Objectives of the section

Provide a comprehensive understanding of the mechanisms underlying happiness, integrating physiological and psychological aspects.

Key topics

BIOLOGICAL FOUNDATIONS OF HAPPINESS - Explores the physiological mechanisms underlying happiness, including sensory input, brain structures, neurotransmitters, hormones, and the peripheral nervous system.

PSYCHOLOGICAL INFLUENCES ON HAPPINESS - Discusses cognitive processes such as cognitive appraisal and their impact on emotional experiences.

Achieving happiness in life is deeply intertwined with the intricate workings of the human body. The generation of emotions and feelings is a symphony orchestrated by a blend of physiological and psychological elements, each playing a crucial role in shaping our inner landscape.

Let's delve into the labyrinth of these intricacies and explore how they harmonize to create our emotional experiences:

Sensory Input - External stimuli or internal cues serve as the catalyst for emotional responses. Our senses act as conduits, channeling information to the brain for interpretation, initiating a cascade of reactions within us.

Brain Structures - At the helm of this process lies the limbic system, a network of structures like the amygdala, hippocampus and hypothalamus. Here, sensory inputs are processed, birthing emotional responses that color our perceptions of the world by initiating appropriate responses involving the release of neurotransmitters.

Neurotransmitters - Chemical messengers called neurotransmitters play a crucial role in regulating and choreographing the dance of our emotions. They transmit signals across synapses (gaps between nerve cells) in the nervous system. They act locally and quickly, influencing the activity of neighboring neurons. Neurotransmitters are primarily involved in communication within the nervous system, regulating functions such as mood, cognition, and muscle movement. Key neurotransmitters related to happiness are:

- *Serotonin* is mainly produced in the brain, particularly in the raphe nuclei and the pineal gland. It is often referred to as the "feel-good" neurotransmitter. It helps regulate mood, appetite, and sleep. Low levels of serotonin have been linked to mood disorders like depression, while higher levels are associated with feelings of happiness and well-being.
- *Dopamine* is synthesized in various areas of the brain, including the substantia nigra and the ventral tegmental area. It is commonly known as the "reward" neurotransmitter. It plays a key role in the brain's reward system, influencing motivation,

pleasure, and reinforcement of behaviors. Increased dopamine activity is associated with feelings of enjoyment and satisfaction.

- *Endorphins* are produced by the pituitary gland and the hypothalamus in the brain, as well as by other tissues throughout the body. They are natural painkillers produced by the body in response to stress or pain. They are often referred to as the body's "natural opioids" because they can induce feelings of euphoria and well-being. Endorphins are released during exercise, laughter, and other activities.
- *Norepinephrine* is both a neurotransmitter and a hormone, often associated with the body's "fight or flight" response to stress. It helps regulate arousal, attention, and focus. In certain situations, increased norepinephrine levels can contribute to feelings of alertness and excitement, which may enhance mood under certain circumstances.

Neurotransmitters modulate neuronal activity within the brain, influencing cognitive processes such as cognitive appraisal.

Cognitive Appraisal - Our interpretations of events wield immense power over our emotional landscape. Cognitive processes, such as memories, attention, and judgment, converge to shape our perceptions, triggering hormonal responses that echo throughout our being.

Hormones - Hormones also influence emotions. Hormones are chemical messengers secreted by glands into the bloodstream, regulating various physiological processes such as growth, metabolism, reproduction, and stress response. They act more slowly than neurotransmitters but have longer-lasting effects due to their systemic distribution. Key hormones related to happiness are:

- *Oxytocin*, known as the "love hormone" or "bonding hormone," is associated with social bonding and trust. Positive social interactions, such as hugging or bonding with loved ones, can trigger oxytocin release. Oxytocin promotes feelings of trust, connection, and emotional bonding.

- *Cortisol*, often referred to as the "stress hormone," cortisol levels increase during periods of stress. Chronic stress and elevated cortisol levels can negatively impact mood and overall well-being.
- *Ghrelin and leptin*, which are involved in regulating hunger and satiety. Imbalances in these hormones can affect mood and energy levels.
- *Endorphins* (again): While also acting as neurotransmitters, endorphins function as hormones when released into the bloodstream. Their role in pain relief and pleasure extends to hormonal regulation, contributing to overall happiness and well-being.

Hormones released into the bloodstream can give feedback to the brain, influencing brain function and emotional responses. Positive experiences, social interactions, and activities like exercise and adequate sleep contribute to the production of these hormones, and the interplay of these hormones creates a complex but interconnected system influencing overall feelings of happiness. Conversely, imbalances or deficiencies in these hormones can contribute to feelings of unhappiness or mood disorders. Regular exercise, healthy eating, stress management, positive social connections, and engaging in rewarding activities are vital for maintaining a healthy balance and well-being.

Peripheral Nervous System - The autonomic nervous system, with its sympathetic and parasympathetic branches, helps regulate physiological responses associated with emotions, such as changes in heart rate, breathing, and perspiration.

The Peripheral Nervous System facilitates communication between the brain and peripheral organs, coordinating physiological responses to sensory input and cognitive appraisal.

Within this intricate web, individual variations emerge, shaped by genetics, environment, and life experiences. Yet, amidst this complexity lies hope - the brain's remarkable ability to adapt and change, sculpting neural pathways toward enduring happiness. To unlock the secrets of the multifaceted gem of happiness, we must embrace the holistic tapestry of our lives:

- *Physical Health*: A sanctuary for the soul, built on the pillars of exercise, rest, and nourishment.
- *Social Connections*: Nurturing relationships with loved ones is the cornerstone of emotional well-being.
- *Purposeful Pursuits*: Setting sail towards meaningful goals guided by our values and passions.
- *Gratitude and Mindfulness*: Cultivating presence and appreciation for life's simple joys.
- *Acts of Kindness*: Extending a hand of compassion and generosity to others.
- *Positive Thinking*: Harnessing the power of optimism to weather life's storms with grace.

In conclusion, our emotions are a fine tissue woven from the threads of physiology, cognition, and environment. By understanding and embracing this intricate dance, we can unlock the gates to enduring happiness and fulfilment in our lives.

6 Who am I and who do I want to be?

"The only thing that will make you happy is being happy with who you are, and not who people think you are."

Goldie Hawn - American actress and producer

"The greatest discovery of all time is that a person can change his future by merely changing his attitude."

Oprah Winfrey - American talk show host, television producer, actress, author, and philanthropist

---

6.1 The Journey of Self-Integration: Navigating the Depths of Human Nature - The "selfishness" model

"To be yourself in a world that is constantly trying to make you something else is the greatest accomplishment."

Ralph Waldo Emerson - American essayist, lecturer, philosopher, and poet.

"Compare yourself to who you were yesterday, not to who someone else is today"

Jordan Peterson - Psychologist, author, and media commentator

Objectives of the section

Explore the journey of self-integration, focusing on how individuals navigate the complexities of human nature, from self-centeredness to interconnectedness, and the evolution of relationships.

Key topics

STAGES OF SELF-INTEGRATION - Describe the progression from self-centeredness to interconnectedness, including five stages. Each stage reflects a nuanced interplay between self-discovery and communal harmony.

THE JOHARI WINDOW - Introduce the Johari Window psychological framework. The text discusses its four quadrants (Open/self, Blind, Hidden, Unknown) and how it aids in understanding self-awareness and fostering meaningful connections.

In the complex web of life, people often focus on themselves, influenced by biology, society, and survival instincts. This self-focus, shaped by thousands of years of adaptation, arises from the basic urge to stay alive. Evolutionarily, prioritizing one's safety was crucial for survival in tough environments.

Moreover, actual societal structures echo this sentiment, urging individuals to carve their paths toward personal fulfilment and success. From cultural expectations to economic systems, the narrative of individual achievement reverberates, shaping aspirations and values from the earliest stages of life. Yet, woven amidst this self-centered narrative lies the undeniable truth of human interconnectedness, including emotional support, companionship, and mutual aid, a truth that transcends the bounds of self-interest, calling us to forge bonds of kinship and collaboration.

As we navigate the labyrinth of existence, we embark on a journey marked by varying degrees of self-awareness and integration with others, including friendships, romantic relationships, and participation in communities and social networks. From the solitary confines of the self to the boundless expanses of interconnectedness, each stage reflects a nuanced interplay between self-discovery and communal harmony. Through nurturing qualities such as empathy, compassion, and a spirit of togetherness, we can develop profound relationships that enhance their own sense of fulfilment and promote the welfare of those in their midst.

In Section 5.1, we explored Maslow's hierarchy of needs, which acts as a guiding light, helping us understand the diverse spectrum of human behavior. It reveals how we navigate our actions driven by self-interest while gradually forming deeper connections with the world around us. Similarly, I wanted to share my perspective on the various stages of individual self-focus, which can be categorized into five phases, each demonstrating a growing sense of association and integration with others. Just like Maslow's hierarchy of needs, the journey from one stage to the next is not a straight path, and the connections between them are complex and influenced by many factors. However, it provides us with a framework for our personal growth and relationships, always reminding us to honor ourselves and our values.

Me

At the onset of this journey inward, as individuals, we find ourselves cocooned within the intricate web of our own identity. Here, the primal urges and basic needs exert a profound influence, shaping the very essence of our existence. It is a stage marked by an intense focus on self-preservation and survival, where our primary concern revolves around fulfilling our most fundamental physiological and safety needs. Every action is driven by the imperative of securing food, shelter, and safety, laying the foundation upon which higher levels of self-awareness and personal growth can later be built.

Me and others

Emerging from the shadow confines of self-absorption, our individual selves tentatively acknowledge the existence of others in our orbit. However, this recognition is often filtered through the lens of personal gain and self-interest. Relationships at this stage are transactional in nature, with the individual forming connections primarily to satisfy our own needs for security, companionship, and validation. Trust is tentative, and interactions are characterized by cautious reciprocity as we navigate the delicate balance between self-preservation and social engagement.

Me for others

As our understanding of interpersonal dynamics deepens, we become increasingly adept at leveraging relationships to serve our own interests, even if this is done unconsciously. This stage is characterized by an approach to social interactions, where others are viewed as tools or resources to be utilized for personal gain. We may then cultivate an image of empathy and altruism to manipulate others into fulfilling their needs while maintaining a careful façade of concern for the well-being of those around us. Despite the apparent focus on self-interest, this stage also involves a keen understanding of social cues and dynamics, allowing us to navigate complex interpersonal relationships with finesse and skill.

Others for me

As our understanding of the environment and interactions with others deepens, a newfound awareness of the power dynamics at play emerges. Leveraging relationships becomes a conscious strategy to fulfill personal needs, marking a return to self-focus albeit with a heightened sophistication. Driven by the desire for uniqueness and distinction, we then strategically utilize others as instruments to achieve our own objectives.

Despite this self-oriented approach, we maintain a veneer of empathy and people-centric behavior, skillfully navigating social dynamics to ensure we are perceived as understanding and considerate. This strategic behavior is underpinned by a comprehensive understanding of others' needs and behaviors, allowing us to wield influence and garner respect while still pursuing our own agenda.

This level can often be described as a phase where we begin to explore the realms of influence and manipulation. While the focus remains on our personal objectives, adeptness at understanding and meeting the needs of others ensures a delicate balance between self-interest and maintaining positive interpersonal relationships.

ME

At the pinnacle of awareness, our focus turns entirely inward, achieving an unparalleled mastery of self and surroundings. This state represents the culmination of a profound journey towards self-actualization, where we transcend the limitations of the ego and attain a sublime understanding of our place in the universe.

Unlike the initial stage where self-awareness was rudimentary or non-existent, at this level, self-awareness reaches its zenith. We become acutely attuned to our own desires, motivations, and innermost workings, fostering a deep sense of introspection and self-reflection.

This heightened state of self-awareness enables us to navigate the complexities of human interactions with unparalleled clarity and grace. Relationships with others become vehicles for personal growth and self-discovery rather than mere instruments for fulfilling needs or desires.

In some cases, we may even experience a profound disconnection between body and soul, a state often associated with highly spiritual or enlightened minds. This experience transcends the confines of the physical realm, offering a glimpse into the deeper truths of existence and the interconnectedness of all beings.

Table 1 delineates the journey through the five states of selfishness, illustrating our evolution as well as our interactions with others. Commencing with a focus on the personal self lays the groundwork for expanding horizons, fostering deeper relationships, and engaging with the external environment in more nuanced ways.

Table 1: The five states of selfishness and the corresponding evolution, including interactions with others

Me	me and others	me for others	Others for me	ME
me	me / Others	Others ↑ me	me ↑ Others	ME

A crucial aspect in navigating this intricate and nonlinear journey is the continual reinforcement of our understanding of both us and the surrounding environment. It is through this understanding that we can effectively integrate new knowledge into our thoughts and personal development. The presence of the unknown adds to the complexity, potentially leading to uncertainty and ambiguity. Therefore, by expanding our awareness and knowledge, we can navigate this journey with greater clarity and purpose. The Johari Window, a psychological framework, serves as a multifaceted lens through which individuals perceive themselves and are perceived by others, serving as a valuable aid in personal self-discovery and development. This model delineates four distinct quadrants, each offering insights into different facets of self-awareness:

- **Open/self**: Aspects known to both the individual and others.
- **Blind**: Traits recognized by others but not acknowledged by the individual.
- **Hidden**: Elements known to the individual but concealed from others.
- **Unknown**: Aspects neither recognized by the individual nor by others.

In the context of self-focus and the journey towards integration with others, the Johari Window highlights the significance of the "*Open/self*" quadrant. Here, we are aware of aspects of us that are also perceptible to others, forming the foundation for authentic interpersonal connections.

However, true integration necessitates an exploration of the "*Hidden*" quadrant, where aspects of the self lie concealed from external view. By courageously revealing these hidden dimensions, we can deepen our relationships, fostering mutual understanding and empathy.

Acknowledging the existence of the "*Blind*" quadrant underscores the importance of soliciting feedback from others. Such insights into our blind spots and areas for personal growth are invaluable, facilitating self-discovery and fostering meaningful connections.

In essence, the Johari Window underscores the dynamic nature of self-awareness and the pivotal role of open communication and mutual disclosure in cultivating rich and fulfilling relationships. This framework reinforces the interconnectedness between self-awareness, interpersonal dynamics, and the broader journey of personal growth and integration.

As we embark on this voyage of self-discovery, we unearth the tools necessary to navigate the currents of existence. The Johari Window, a prism illuminating the facets of self-awareness, serves as a guidepost in this journey. From the open expanse of known truths to the hidden recesses of untapped potential, each quadrant beckons exploration and revelation. Through introspection and mutual disclosure, we will forge connections that transcend the boundaries of our self, enriching our lives and those of others.

In life's grand orchestra, our personal journey blends with the rhythms of community, resonating throughout history. As we navigate life's twists and turns, we create a unique identity that is shaped by both self-discovery and our connections with others. May this journey bring us comfort, fulfilment, and the warmth of human connection.

The remainder of this section will delve into the pivotal elements that underpin our self-concept, aiding in the exploration of our personal identity and facilitating our growth as we engage with others, whether it be within societal settings, intimate relationships, or professional environments.

6.2   Understanding Your Roots

"The most terrifying thing is to accept oneself completely."

Carl Jung - Swiss psychiatrist, psychoanalyst

"Knowing yourself is the beginning of all wisdom."

Aristotle - Greek philosopher

Objectives of the section

Start with self-discovery. Understand your strengths, weaknesses, interests, and passions. This will reinforce self-awareness and will provide a foundation for the subsequent steps.

Key topics

PAST EXPERIENCES - Your past experiences, both positive and negative, contribute to your understanding of yourself. They can inform your strengths, weaknesses, preferences, and fears.

EXTERNAL INFLUENCES - External factors such as culture, family, peers, education, and society as a whole impact your identity and shape your values, beliefs, and behaviors.

EMOTIONS AND FEELINGS - Emotions and feelings provide valuable insights into your inner world. They reflect your responses to experiences and external stimuli, indicating what matters to you and what triggers certain reactions.

During my early years, I resided in a small, serene town in Switzerland, living with my parents and siblings in a nice house surrounded by a small garden where I used to play when the sun was shining. Timid and contemplative, I navigated the twists and turns of growing up with caution, yearning to explore beyond my familiar surroundings but uncertain of where I truly belonged. Yet amidst my hesitations, I found solace in the embrace of friendship, a sanctuary where I could be myself without inhibition or doubt, whether at school, playing soccer, or inventing great stories within the Roman ruins surrounding the town. From my earliest days, I cultivated deep bonds with a select few kindred souls with whom I felt understood and safe. Together, we were able to discover the world without fearing being confronted by the harsh reality of the outer world.

But at the tender age of seven, my world was rocked by the harsh hand of fate. Torn away from all I held dear, I embarked on a journey to a foreign town as my parents had to move for professional reasons. I became a stranger in a land of unfamiliar faces and customs and lost all the connections that had taken me years to build. Trying to maintain this past safe cocoon, I communicated for several months with my former friends, sending and receiving vibrant letters and drawings, which, even if providing me with a sense of happiness, prevented me from integrating into my new home place. Lost amidst a sea of strangers, I felt adrift, a vessel without a guiding star tossed in turbulent waters. Desperate to reclaim the familiarity of my former life, I erected walls around my heart, shielding myself from the ache of separation and longing. Yet beneath my stoic facade, the heart of a child continued to beat with the rhythm of yearning—for connection, for acceptance, for the simple pleasure of being seen and understood. I was withdrawn, letting nothing show on the outside but suffering from loneliness and irrational fears deep down inside.

It was not until years later, as I stood on the precipice of adulthood that I came to recognize the profound influence of my childhood. Engaging in deep introspection, I realized the pivotal role all these events played in shaping my identity, my sense of belonging, and how they made me the man I had become. With this newfound insight, inspired by "The Child In You: The Breakthrough Method for Bringing Out Your Authentic Self" by Stefanie Stahl, a renowned German psychotherapist, I embarked on a journey of self-discovery and healing. Delving into the depths of my inner child, I confronted past wounds, reconnected with my authentic self, and embraced vulnerability and emotional expression. Armed with the knowledge that I was deserving of love and belonging, I stepped boldly into the world, starting to confront all my fears and anxieties, determined to demolish the walls I had built to protect myself from the outside world.

I did not realize that I was embarking on a long and difficult journey that would take me through peaks and valleys, revealing my deepest emotions and feelings, and would bring me to uncover who I really was. This was the starting point of my discovery of happiness, which I, at one point, considered I was not allowed to reach.

Through reflection on key past events, impactful experiences, significant relationships, and emotional responses, you can identify recurring patterns and themes that shape your understanding of yourself. By analyzing how these events have influenced your development and perspectives, you can gain clarity on your core values and aspirations for the future.

Your journey of self-discovery begins with a deep dive into your past, aiming to understand the events that have shaped you, the environments that have influenced you, the people who have walked alongside you, and the emotions that have colored your experiences. By evaluating these key elements, you gain insight into your personal values and what truly matters to you. As you piece together the puzzle of your life story, you uncover the threads that weave through your identity, guiding you towards a clearer understanding of your dreams and wishes. This process of introspection and reflection empowers you to articulate your personal meaning in life, creating a foundation for living authentically and purposefully. Through consistency and impact, your journey of self-discovery becomes a transformative exploration of identity, values, and aspirations, illuminating the path towards personal fulfilment.

Remember that your journey of self-discovery is unique to you, and it is okay to take the time to explore and understand yourself at your own pace.

6.2.1 Unearthing Defining Moments

Embark on your journey of self-discovery by focusing on significant events that have left an imprint on your life, whether positively or negatively. Reflect on moments that have evoked profound emotions and sentiments within you, spanning childhood, adolescence, and adulthood. These could encompass milestones such as completing your education, relocating to a new city, commencing a fresh career, entering into marriage, coping with the loss of a loved one, or surmounting personal hurdles. It is imperative to approach this process with full openness, embracing every memory, as both moments of joy and sorrow hold crucial insights into understanding your essence and motivations. To assist in this endeavor, consider categorizing these events under various themes:

1. Personal achievement
2. Major change
3. Health crisis/accident
4. Economic downturn
5. Social event
6. Party/celebration
7. Sport event
8. Vacation/travel
9. Life transition (marriage, parenthood....)
10. Personal loss (death, divorce, ...)

Identify 3 to 5 key events as a starting point and refer to the related cards here under.

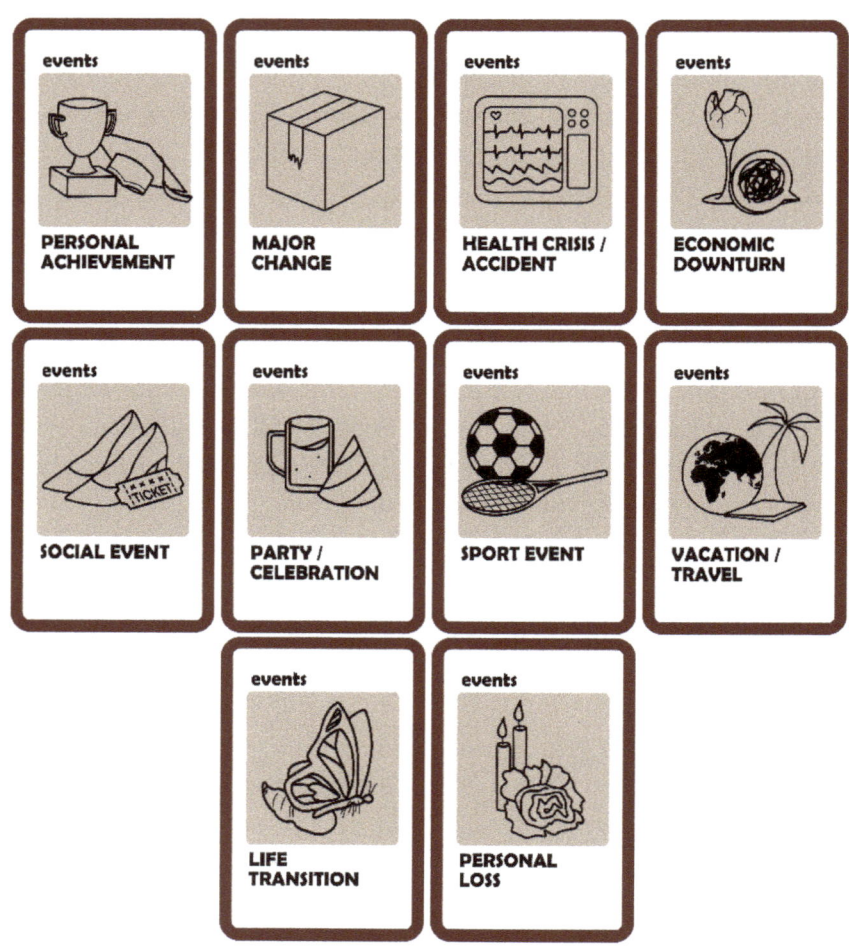

This will then be refined and detailed to make them more precise and clarify what they triggered in you and why.

My self-discovery - Defining events

Here, I delineate three pivotal moments in my life, which I have recognized as defining after reflecting on my past experiences.

First pivotal moment - Major change

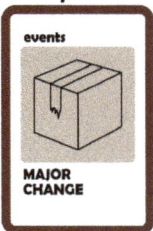

From the outset, my journey has been one marked by a profound divergence from the norm, defined by an innate depth of emotion and sensitivity that set me apart from my peers. In a world where societal expectations dictated that boys should exude strength and resilience, I found myself grappling with an inner turmoil I dared not reveal. This inner conflict propelled me on a relentless quest for truth and understanding, urging me to dissect and interpret the complexities of life while navigating the turbulent seas of intense emotion. It was not until later that I recognized these experiences mirrored the intellectual and emotional overexcitability identified by Dabrowski and Piechowski.

Physically, the toll was palpable – from the stomachaches to the involuntary blushes, even grappling with the weight of existential concerns like death and depression. These manifestations were not easily concealed, often subjecting me to ridicule and mockery, amplifying my sense of vulnerability.

For the first seven years of my life, my familial support and stable surroundings provided a semblance of control over these challenges, fostering close friendships and a nurturing environment both at home and school. However, the equilibrium shattered when circumstances forced a relocation, stripping away the protective layers I had painstakingly built.

Caught in the throes of unfamiliarity, I found myself retreating further into isolation, severing ties with the joys of life – the wonder, the beauty, the compassion, and the creative spark dimmed beneath the weight of sadness and anxiety. Yet, in my solitude, I shielded my anguish from my parents, unwilling to burden them with the truth, inadvertently denying myself the solace of their support.

In the silence of my struggle, I yearned for recognition, for someone to acknowledge the turmoil festering within. Yet, as the facade of normalcy persisted, my parents remained unaware, leaving me to navigate the tempest alone, bereft of the empathy and understanding I so desperately craved.

Second pivotal moment - Life transition

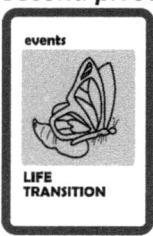

My foray into the professional world commenced upon the completion of my PhD, thrusting me into the unfamiliar terrain of corporate life. Initially, I embraced the novelty with fervor, relishing in the acquisition of new experiences, skills, and capabilities. Recognized as an engaged and high-performing employee with vast potential for growth, I embarked on a journey of self-evolution and empowerment.

With each stride forward, fueled by burgeoning knowledge and self-assurance, my optimism swelled, buoyed by the prospect of effecting real change. However, as I began to articulate my opinions with increasing candor and transparency, anticipating acknowledgment for my sincerity and dedication to improvement, I was blindsided by the harsh reality that unfiltered truth was not always met with gratitude. Instead, I found myself accused of communication deficiencies, a revelation that forced me to confront the incongruence between professed values and actual practices.

Navigating the treacherous waters of political expectations, I grappled with the realization that discretion often eclipses transparency in professional settings, a bitter pill to swallow. As the chasm widened between rhetoric and reality, frustration burgeoned within me, festering into simmering resentment and indignation. This emotional turbulence drove me to escalate my directness, inadvertently leading to allegations of harassment leveled against me by a close colleague.

Though I managed to vindicate myself and catalyze the replacement of my superior, the pervasive internal discord within the organization proved insurmountable. Despite the apparent solidarity of colleagues who supported my viewpoints in private discussions, the toxic atmosphere rendered my continued presence untenable. Thus, with a heavy heart, I bid farewell to the organization, a casualty of the dissonance between principles and practices.

Third pivotal moment - Personal loss

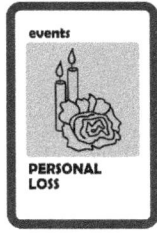

In my twenties, a subtle realization dawned upon me – the recognition of my own worth in the eyes of others, prompting a tentative emergence from the protective confines of my shell and the initial construction of self-assurance. Although I failed to grasp at the time that this was merely the nascent stage of my journey towards self-discovery, I reveled in the newfound joys of life, finding profound happiness in the companionship of the woman who would later become my wife, an anchor in my journey of personal growth.

For the ensuing fifteen years, I basked in what I believed to be my long-awaited stability – marriage, two beautiful daughters, the construction of a home, and success in my career. Embracing the comforting illusion of normalcy, I was enveloped by waves of gratitude, contentment, and tranquility. Yet, amidst these positive emotions, I failed to recognize that this was but a single chapter in the grand narrative of my existence. Deep within, a gnawing sense of discontent simmered, ignored in the bliss of the moment. Underestimating the perpetual nature of self-discovery, I unwittingly drifted towards a precipice, ultimately culminating in a divorce and a prolonged period of introspection, grappling with the weight of sadness, guilt, and regret.

In the crucible of solitude, the amicable rapport maintained with my ex-wife served as a beacon, illuminating the shadows of my inner turmoil. It was during this time of reflection that I came to realize the multifaceted tapestry of life and the immutable truth articulated by Eugene Sandow, German bodybuilder and showman – "Life is movement. Once you stop moving, you're dead. Choose life." Though our paths diverged, I understood that this pivotal juncture had sculpted the very core of my being, a testament to the ceaseless evolution inherent in the human experience.

6.2.2   Influence of Environments

Consider the settings and circumstances surrounding the chosen events, observing how they shaped your experiences and viewpoints. The context in which these events unfolded is crucial, as it influences the emotions and sentiments involved, facilitating the consolidation of personal motivations, beliefs, and values. Examples of environments pertinent to your pivotal events may include:

1. Home
2. School
3. Workplace
4. Outdoor space
5. Shopping malls/markets
6. Social events or gatherings
7. Restaurants/cafes
8. Recreational areas (such as gym facilities, parks, or beaches)
9. Public transport
10. Public facilities

By examining the interplay between your experiences and the environments in which they occurred, you gain deeper insights into the factors shaping your journey and contributing to your personal growth. Link each event with the related environment and match the related cards together.

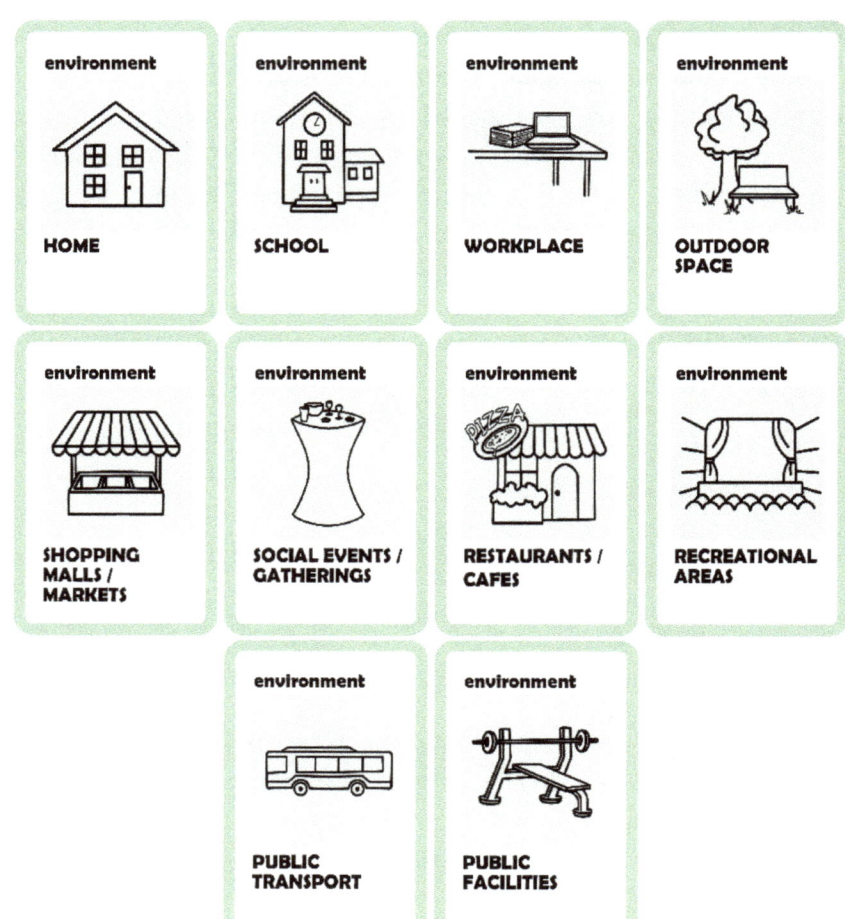

Once the events are distinctly identified and linked with their respective environments, the subsequent crucial step is to ascertain the individuals who were associated or connected with them.

My self-discovery – Environments

My journey of self-discovery revolves around various pivotal life events, as outlined in Section 6.2.1, each deeply intertwined with specific environments.

First pivotal moment - Major change

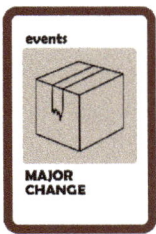

Event description - Relocating at a young age disrupted stability, causing isolation and inner turmoil. Despite supportive familial and friendship ties initially, the new environment brought feelings of sadness and anxiety as the individual grappled with intense emotions alone.

Key involved environments

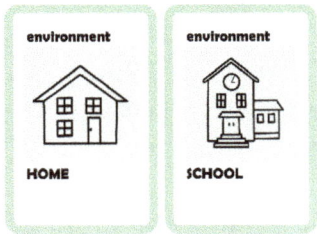

- Initial home: Initially provided stability and familial support.
- Initial school: Nurturing environment fostering close friendships.
- New Location – Both home and school: Unfamiliarity and unsettling surroundings.

Second pivotal moment - Life transition

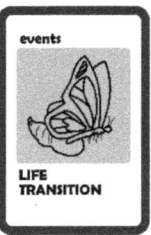

Event description - Transitioning into the professional world after completing a PhD led to initial optimism but later frustration due to workplace practices not aligned with professed values. Accusations of harassment further exacerbated internal conflict, ultimately leading to departure from the toxic environment.

Key involved environment

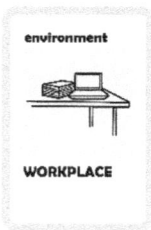

- Workplace: Initially perceived as a place of growth and empowerment, but which evolved into a politically charged and incongruent place with professed values.

Third pivotal moment - Personal loss

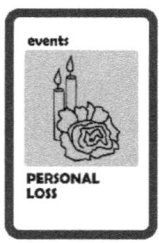

Event description - A stable period in adulthood was shattered by divorce, leading to introspection and self-discovery. Amidst feelings of sadness, regret, and guilt, maintaining an amicable relationship with the ex-wife and prioritizing familial bonds highlighted the importance of growth and acceptance in the face of personal loss.

Key involved environments

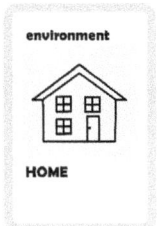

- Home: Initially a haven of stability and happiness, which became a space for introspection and reflection after divorce.

6.2.3   Significance of Relationships

Based on the selected events and their associated environments, identify the individuals who were involved in the related relationships, as they likely played significant roles in shaping your life journey. These individuals could include family members, friends, mentors, romantic partners, or colleagues. Begin by reflecting on how these relationships have influenced your beliefs, values, and behaviors during the corresponding events. The types of individuals involved may encompass:

1. Parents
2. Siblings
3. Friends
4. Partner
5. Children
6. Teacher
7. Boss
8. Colleague
9. Therapist/coach
10. Self/alone

By examining the impact of these relationships, you gain insights into the dynamics that have influenced your personal development and trajectory. Link each event with the involved people and match the related cards together.

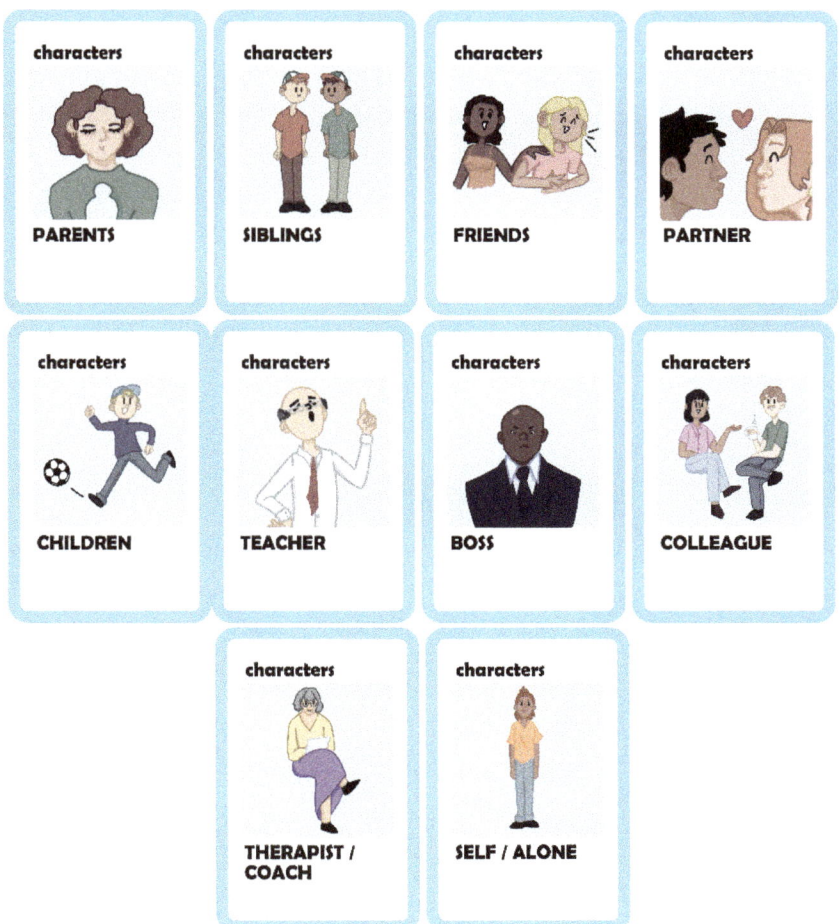

The ultimate step involves pinpointing the emotions and sentiments that were elicited by the identified events with as much precision as possible. This phase can be particularly challenging as it may resurface difficult and painful memories. However, it also presents an opportunity to recollect uplifting moments that may have faded from memory.

Therefore, it is crucial to allocate sufficient time to this phase of the self-discovery process, allowing yourself to fully absorb any positive or negative personal impacts. Additionally, take the opportunity to reflect on the implications and effects these emotions have had on your inner self.

My self-discovery – People and relationships

Returning to significant moments in my life, the presence and impact of key individuals and relationships were paramount.

First pivotal moment - Major change

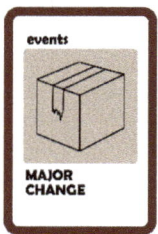

Event description - Relocating at a young age disrupted stability, causing isolation and inner turmoil. Despite supportive familial and friendship ties initially, the new environment brought feelings of sadness and anxiety as the individual grappled with intense emotions alone.

Key involved people/relationships

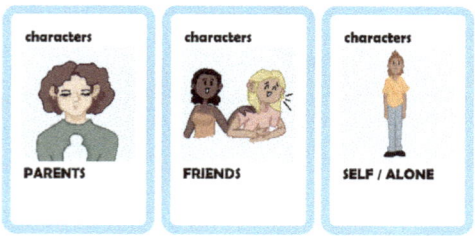

- Parents: Initially supportive but unaware of the inner turmoil.
- Friends: Provided companionship and joy before the relocation.
- Self: Struggling with intense emotions and a sense of isolation.

Second pivotal moment – Life transition

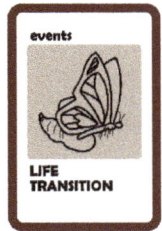

Event description – Transitioning into the professional world after completing a PhD led to initial optimism but later frustration due to workplace practices not aligned with professed values. Accusations of harassment further exacerbated internal conflict, ultimately leading to departure from the toxic environment.

Key involved people/relationships:

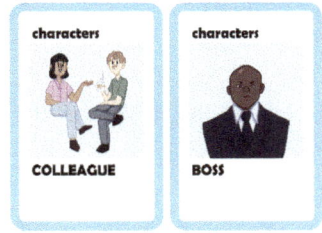

- Colleagues: Some were supportive, but others contributed to the toxic atmosphere and made some accusations of harassment, leading to internal conflict.
- Boss: Initially considered as a mentor, but later became a source of frustration.

Third pivotal moment - Personal loss

Event description - A stable period in adulthood was shattered by divorce, leading to introspection and self-discovery. Amidst feelings of sadness, regret, and guilt, maintaining an amicable relationship with the ex-wife and prioritizing familial bonds highlighted the importance of growth and acceptance in the face of personal loss.

Key involved people/relationships

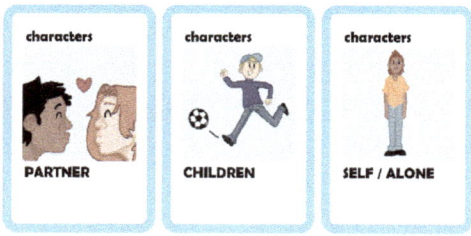

- Ex-Wife: Maintained amicable rapport, serving as a guide during introspection.
- Children: Presence highlighted the importance of family despite divorce.
- Self: Experienced personal growth and acceptance through introspection.

6.2.4   Delving into Emotions

For a comprehensive understanding of your emotional responses to the chosen events, delve deeply into the feelings that accompanied them, considering both the environment in which they transpired and the relationships involved. Reflect on how you felt during moments of triumph, disappointment, affection, betrayal, or uncertainty. Acknowledge the spectrum of emotions you have experienced and how they have influenced your perspective. You can select from a range of positive and negative emotions from the lists below.

Positive Feelings

1. Joy
2. Gratitude
3. Love
4. Serenity
5. Hope
6. Contentment
7. Excitement
8. Confidence
9. Pride
10. Inspiration

Negative Feelings

1. Anger
2. Sadness
3. Despair
4. Disgust
5. Guilt
6. Frustration
7. Envy
8. Anxiety
9. Regret
10. Shame

By recognizing and exploring these emotions, you gain deeper insight into their impact on your perceptions and beliefs, fostering a clearer understanding of your emotional landscape. Link each event with the related feelings and match the related cards together.

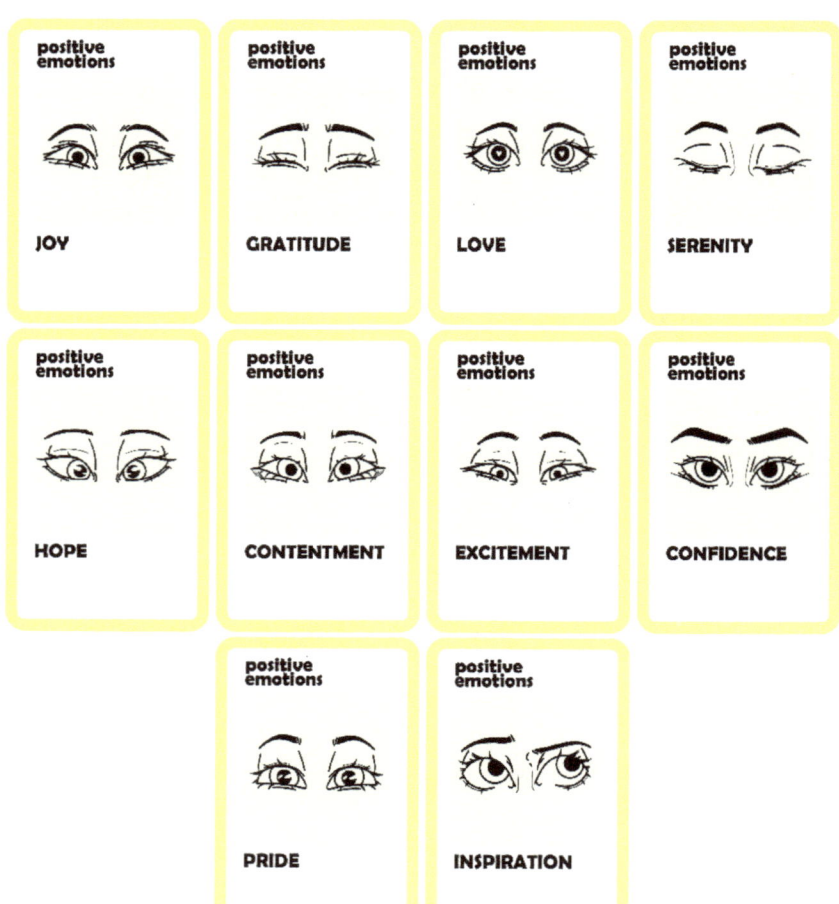

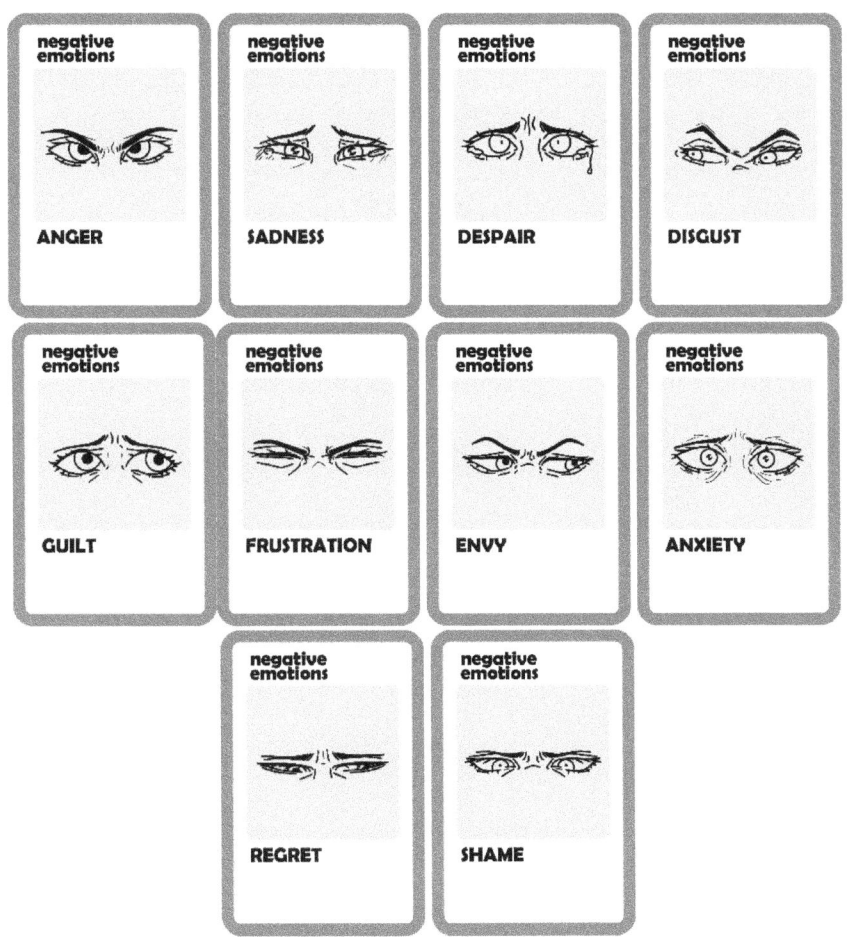

By integrating the associated emotions and feelings with the events, alongside the environments and individuals involved, you assemble a curated collection of experiences crucial to defining your identity. These experiences serve as foundational elements that enable you to comprehend your motivations, values, and principles. They become the building blocks and adhesive as you construct your future self, leveraging these insights to navigate your path forward with clarity and purpose.

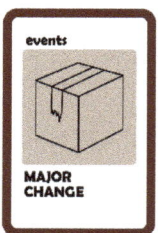

My self-discovery – Feelings and emotions

In contemplating my significant life events, I have discerned both positive and negative emotions that accompanied me during these periods.

First pivotal moment - Major change

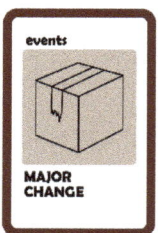

Event description - Relocating at a young age disrupted stability, causing isolation and inner turmoil. Despite supportive familial and friendship ties initially, the new environment brought feelings of sadness and anxiety as the individual grappled with intense emotions alone.

Key related emotions

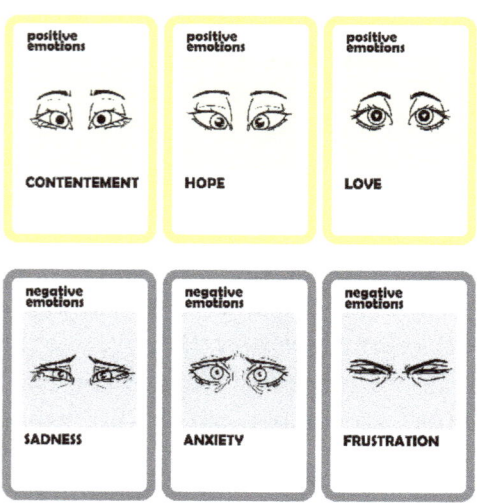

- Positive: Contentment (before relocation), hope (for understanding), love (from family).
- Negative: Sadness (due to isolation), anxiety (in unfamiliar surroundings), frustration (at being misunderstood).

Second pivotal moment - Life transition

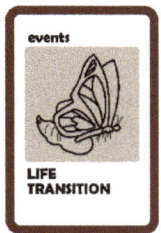

Event description - Transitioning into the professional world after completing a PhD led to initial optimism but later frustration due to workplace practices not aligned with professed values. Accusations of harassment further exacerbated internal conflict, ultimately leading to departure from the toxic environment.

Key related emotions

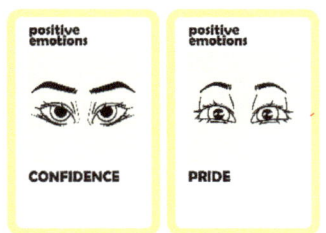 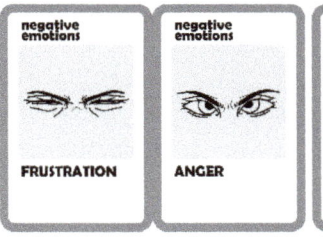

- Positive: Confidence (initially), pride (in effecting change).
- Negative: Frustration (at incongruent values), anger (towards workplace dynamics), anxiety (about future career prospects).

Third pivotal moment - Personal loss

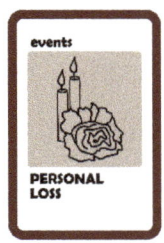

Event description - A stable period in adulthood was shattered by divorce, leading to introspection and self-discovery. Amidst feelings of sadness, regret, and guilt, maintaining an amicable relationship with the ex-wife and prioritizing familial bonds highlighted the importance of growth and acceptance in the face of personal loss.

Key related emotions

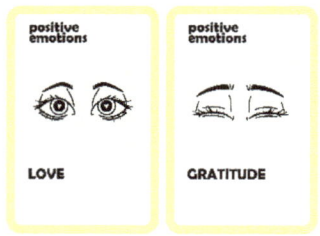 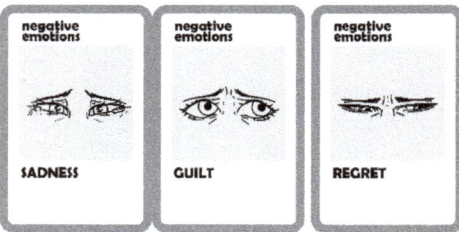

- Positive: Love (for family), gratitude (for past stability).
- Negative: Sadness (at a loss of marriage), guilt (over missed opportunities), regret (for not recognizing inner discontent).

6.2.5 Strengthening Selfhood for the Journey

Now that you have gained a comprehensive understanding of the pivotal past events, impactful experiences, significant relationships, and emotional responses that have shaped you, it is crucial to delve into how these occurrences have molded your growth and perspective.

Connect deeply with the emotions and feelings they evoked. Did they usher in moments of joy, sorrow, growth, or transformation? Take this opportunity to reflect on the lessons learned and conduct an initial analysis of the insights gleaned from each experience.

This entails, in particular:

- *Identification of patterns and themes* - Delve into your past experiences to uncover any recurring patterns or themes. Are there common threads that intertwine certain events or relationships? Recognizing these patterns can offer valuable insight into your core values, interests, and priorities.
- *Extraction of Personal Values* - Through introspection, distil the values that hold utmost significance to you. Consider the guiding principles that have shaped your decisions and actions over time. These values may encompass integrity, resilience, compassion, authenticity, or the pursuit of knowledge.
- *Clarification of dreams and aspirations* - With a deeper comprehension of your past experiences and values, envision your dreams and aspirations for the future. What are the goals and ambitions that resonate most deeply with you? Reflect on the kind of life you aspire to create for yourself and the legacy you aim to leave behind.

This introspective journey aligns your past experiences with your personal sense of purpose in life, paving the way for a more deliberate and gratifying path forward rooted in authenticity and meaning. It serves as a crucial foundation as you progress to the next steps, which involve delineating your personal values, life principles, and, ultimately, your key life objectives and dreams. This is the focus of the rest of Section 6.

6.3   Unveiling Personal Values

Objectives of the section

Once you have a clearer sense of who you are, identify and prioritize your core values. Your values will shape your goals and guide your actions.

Key topics

SELF REFLECTION - Take time to reflect on your core beliefs, what matters most to you, and the principles you want to govern your life.

IDENTIFY CORE VALUES – Determine your core values. These are the fundamental beliefs that are most important to you. Examples include integrity, honesty, compassion, resilience, and authenticity.

PRIORITIZE KEY VALUES - Arrange your values in order of importance. This helps you understand which values are non-negotiable and central to your decision-making.

One example of someone known for his strong values and how they impacted their actions and lives is Mahatma Gandhi.

Gandhi's unwavering commitment to nonviolence and truth, known as "satyagraha," profoundly shaped his actions and life. His values were deeply rooted in his upbringing and experiences, including his time in South Africa, where he faced discrimination and injustice.

One concrete example of Gandhi's strong values in action is the Salt March of 1930. In protest of British salt taxes, which disproportionately affected India's poor, Gandhi embarked on a 240-mile journey from his ashram to the coastal town of Dandi. Despite facing arrests and violent opposition, Gandhi and thousands of followers peacefully marched to the sea, where they symbolically produced salt by evaporating seawater.

This act of civil disobedience captured the world's attention and became a turning point in India's struggle for independence. Gandhi's commitment to his values of nonviolence and truth inspired millions to join the fight against British colonial rule, ultimately leading to India's independence in 1947.

Throughout his life, Gandhi's values guided his actions, from his advocacy for the rights of marginalized communities to his efforts to promote religious harmony and social justice. His commitment to truth and nonviolence not only transformed India but also inspired movements for civil rights and social change around the world.

Gandhi's story serves as a powerful example of how strong values can impact not only individual actions but also the course of history. His unwavering commitment to his principles continues to inspire generations to stand up for justice, equality, and truth.

Another notable example of a woman known for her strong values and how they impacted her actions and life is Malala Yousafzai.

Malala's unwavering commitment to education, equality, and human rights has defined her remarkable journey from a young activist to a global symbol of courage and resilience. Growing up in Pakistan's Swat Valley, Malala was an outspoken advocate for girls' education in defiance of the Taliban's oppressive regime.

One concrete example of Malala's strong values in action is her advocacy for girls' education, which began at a young age. Despite facing threats and violence from the Taliban, Malala continued to speak out against the ban on girls attending school, even documenting her experiences anonymously for the BBC.

In 2012, at the age of 15, Malala survived an assassination attempt by the Taliban, who targeted her for her activism. Rather than succumbing to fear, Malala emerged from the attack with an even stronger determination to fight for the rights of girls to receive an education.

Following her recovery, Malala continued her advocacy on a global scale, co-founding the Malala Fund with her father to promote girls' education around the world. Through her powerful speeches, writings, and activism, Malala has become an influential voice for the millions of girls denied access to education due to poverty, conflict, and discrimination.

Malala's values of courage, perseverance, and compassion have not only shaped her own life but have also inspired millions of people worldwide. In 2014, she became the youngest-ever recipient of the Nobel Peace Prize in recognition of her extraordinary efforts to promote education and empower girls.

Despite facing immense challenges and adversity, Malala's unwavering commitment to her values has enabled her to overcome obstacles and make a profound impact on the world. Her story serves as a powerful reminder of the transformative power of strong values and the importance of standing up for what is right, even in the face of daunting odds.

The concept of "value" encompasses a multitude of meanings, spanning from moral principles to worth and usefulness. In the realm of personal identity, it often speaks to one's core beliefs, priorities, and what holds significance or meaning in their life. Recognizing and understanding these values is pivotal in navigating decisions and offering a compass for purposeful living.

For individuals, values serve as the bedrock for discerning what matters most. Clarity in values, coupled with an awareness of their implications, aids in making decisions consistent with one's principles. This fosters a sense of purpose and contributes to personal growth and well-being. Moreover, shared values form the basis of connections with like-minded individuals, laying the groundwork for relationships and community. Such alignment facilitates finding fulfilment and contentment, whether in professional or personal spheres, supporting the journey towards happiness.

Our values reflect our environment and immediate influences and experiences during the first years of our life. Influencing factors include:

- *Family Influence* - Family upbringing and the values instilled by parents or caregivers significantly impact an individual's moral and ethical beliefs.
- *Cultural Background* - Cultural norms, traditions, and societal values can shape an individual's perspectives and values.
- *Education and Environment* - Formal education, exposure to diverse environments, and interactions with different people can broaden perspectives and shape values.
- *Media and Society* - Media, including books, movies, and social media, can influence values by portraying certain behaviors or ideals.
- *Personal Reflection* - Through introspection and self-discovery, individuals can consciously reflect on their beliefs, refining and solidifying their values over time.

During a person's life, values evolve dynamically as we encounter new experiences and gain a deeper understanding of ourselves and of the world around them. This evolution is impacted by:

- *Personal life Experiences* - Significant life events, positive and negative, challenges and successes contribute to the development and refinement of values, influencing what one considers important.
- *Changing Priorities* - Shifts in personal priorities, such as career changes, starting a family, or reaching certain life milestones, can influence values and what one deems important.
- *Maturity and Wisdom* - As individuals mature, they may gain a deeper understanding of themselves and the world, prompting a re-evaluation and refinement of their values.
- *Learning and Education* - Continuous learning and exposure to new ideas can broaden perspectives, leading to a reconsideration and evolution of values.
- *Cultural Shifts* - Societal changes, cultural shifts, and evolving norms can impact individual values, prompting adaptation to align with the evolving collective ethos.
- *Self-Reflection* - Intentional self-reflection allows individuals to question and reassess their values, fostering personal growth and development.

Adaptability and openness to new experiences are essential for the evolution of values over time. It is a dynamic process that reflects the ongoing journey of self-discovery and personal development. In summary, personal values represent what holds the utmost importance, motivating and guiding our actions. To aid in identifying these values, consider the qualities here as potential examples of personal values:

- *Integrity* - Upholding honesty and ethical/moral principles in all aspects of life. This also involves building and maintaining trust in relationships.
- *Respect* - Treating others with consideration, regardless of differences, and valuing diverse perspectives. Understanding and sharing the feelings of others.
- *Responsibility* - Taking accountability for one's actions, decisions, and commitments.

- *Compassion* - Demonstrating empathy, kindness, and consideration toward others. Providing assistance, especially in times of need.
- *Courage* - Facing challenges and difficult situations with bravery and determination. Advocating for what is right, even in the face of opposition.
- *Authenticity* - Being true to oneself, expressing individuality and maintaining genuineness in thoughts, actions, and relationships.
- *Gratitude* - Recognizing, appreciating, and expressing thanks for the positive aspects of life.
- *Open-mindedness* - Willingness to consider new ideas, perspectives, opinions, and experiences. Adapting to change.
- *Equality* - Believing in fairness and treating everyone with equal value and opportunities. Advocating for equal rights.
- *Resilience* - Bouncing back from setbacks and adapting positively to adversity, challenges, and change. Persisting in the face of difficulties.

Represented by the cards here under:

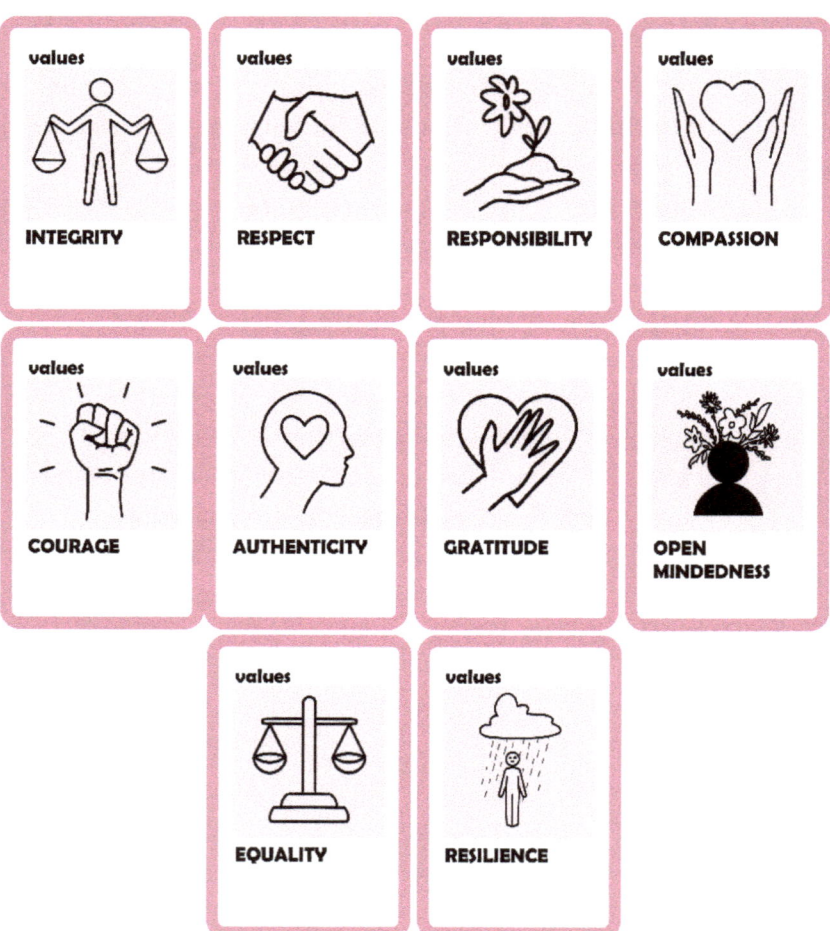

Identifying and prioritizing specific personal values can serve as a compass for decision-making and behaviors, thus shaping one's overall approach to life and fostering fulfilment and purpose.

6.3.1 Exploring Inner Values

To determine your personal values, it is important to reflect on past experiences that brought you fulfilment, consider what aspects of life make you truly happy, and identify principles you naturally prioritize. Engaging in self-discovery through introspection can help unveil your true personal values.

You can then leverage on the key events you identified in your life and what they meant for you or triggered in you, supported by the visuals provided by the cards you selected when describing these in Section 6.2. Try journaling about these moments and how you felt when you experienced them. When did you feel most alive or satisfied? What did trigger the strongest emotions in you? Assess patterns in your interests, behaviors, and choices. In addition, ask yourself what qualities you admire in others. Exploring these aspects can provide clarity on your core values.

Examine positive experiences for common themes and feelings, identifying values that contributed to your happiness. Similarly, analyze negative experiences to pinpoint values that were compromised or clashed. This reflection can offer insights into your core values.

My Guiding Values

Upon deep personal reflection, drawing from past experiences, I have pinpointed certain values that resonate deeply within me, steering the course of my actions and decisions. These values are intricate blends of those introduced here above.

Justice and fairness

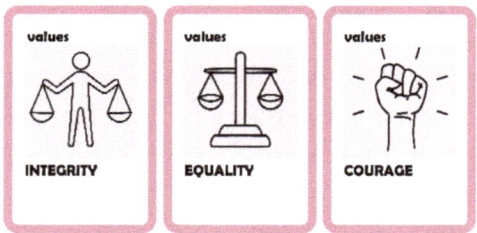

Justice and fairness have been guiding lights throughout my journey, deeply intertwined with my personal experiences and the profound transformations they have triggered. From the tender age of childhood innocence to the complexities of adult life, I have grappled with the visceral impact of unfairness, each instance etching its mark upon my soul.

In the cocoon of my youth, I keenly felt the sting of injustice as societal norms clashed with my inner truth. The upheaval of relocation brought me into unfamiliar terrain, where the expectations of conformity conflicted with my innate sensitivity. Despite the facade of normalcy, the silence surrounding my struggles echoed with the injustice of unacknowledged pain, leaving me to navigate the tempest alone.

As I ventured into the professional realm, the dissonance between professed values and practiced norms became glaringly apparent. My commitment to transparency and honesty collided with a corporate culture steeped in discretion, where unfiltered truth was met with resistance. The allegations of harassment I faced served as a stark reminder of the injustice inherent in a system that prioritizes silence over integrity, leaving me to confront the repercussions of speaking truth to power.

Through the crucible of these experiences, my commitment to justice and fairness has only deepened, anchoring me in moments of doubt and uncertainty. Each trial has reinforced the importance of advocating for equity and confronting injustice, whether in the boardroom or the confines of my own heart. Despite the scars I carry, I remain steadfast in my belief that the pursuit of justice is not merely a noble ideal but a deeply personal imperative, guiding me ever onward on the journey toward a more equitable future.

Respect

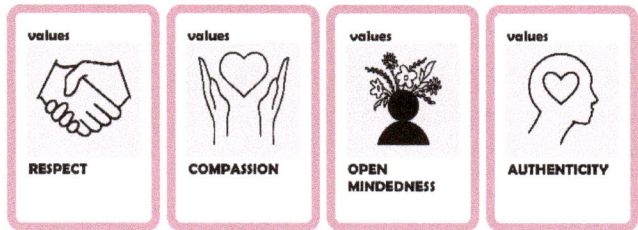

Respect is not just a concept; it is a guiding principle that is woven deeply into the fabric of my life, shaped by the highs and lows of my journey. It is about honoring the intrinsic worth of each person, regardless of our differences, and creating spaces where everyone's voice is heard and valued.

Reflecting on my experiences, respect has been both a beacon of light and a shield against the storms. In the turbulence of my early years, fighting with inner turmoil and societal expectations, I longed for someone to see beyond the surface and respect the depth of my struggles. It was a yearning for recognition, for empathy, for the simple acknowledgment that my journey was valid despite not conforming to norms. This echoes the essence of respect – embracing the uniqueness of each individual, even amidst adversity.

Transitioning into the corporate world brought its own set of challenges, where the clash between transparency and discretion tested the bounds of respect. I learned the hard way that honesty, though valuable, must be tempered with tact and sensitivity. Respect became not just about speaking my truth but also about listening with an open heart to others' perspectives, recognizing the richness that diversity brings to the table.

In the aftermath of personal loss, respect took on a new dimension – one of mutual understanding and acceptance. Despite the pain of divorce, there remained a profound respect for the shared history and the journey that led us to part ways. It was a testament to the enduring bond forged through respect – a recognition of each other's worth and a commitment to honoring our individual paths, even as they diverged.

So, as I navigate life's twists and turns, I strive to cultivate a culture of respect in every interaction, drawing strength from the lessons learned along the way. It is about seeing the humanity in each person, embracing our differences, and forging connections built on a foundation of mutual understanding and empathy.

Trust

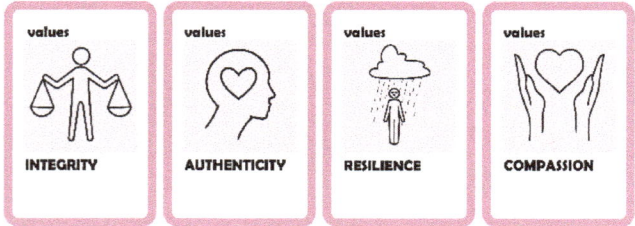

Trust is a bedrock in my life, woven intricately with threads of reliability, integrity, and honesty. It is the steady hand of my family's support during the tumultuous relocation of my childhood, offering a sanctuary amidst the storm of change. Trust lays the foundation for meaningful connections, anchoring me in authenticity and resilience as I navigate life's peaks and valleys.

Yet, trust is not invulnerable. It can fracture, leaving behind jagged edges of betrayal and disillusionment. I felt the sharp sting of betrayal when accusations of harassment were levelled against me by a close colleague, casting doubt on the authenticity of the relationships I held dear. In that moment of reckoning, trust crumbled like sand slipping through my fingers, leaving me grappling with feelings of indignation and resentment.

But amidst the ruins of broken trust, there emerged a beacon of hope – the unwavering trust shared between my ex-wife and me during the upheaval of our divorce. Despite the dissolution of our marriage, our commitment to honesty and mutual respect remained unwavering, a testament to the enduring power of trust even in the face of adversity.

Through the crucible of betrayal, I learned that rebuilding trust requires patience, empathy, and a willingness to extend grace. Just as I sought understanding and empathy during my moments of vulnerability, so too do I strive to cultivate an environment of trust and authenticity in my interactions with others. Trust, I have discovered, is not just a concept but a lived experience shaped by the flow of life's journey.

Personal Development and Challenges

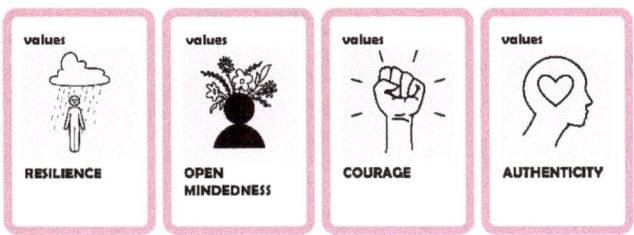

Personal growth is a journey woven intricately with the threads of my own experiences, a narrative that unfolds through moments of profound change and unyielding challenges. It is about more than just accumulating knowledge; it is a relentless pursuit of understanding and self-awareness that has been ingrained in me since the earliest days of my fight with inner turmoil and sensitivity.

From the tender age of seven, when my world was uprooted by relocation, I learned the importance of not settling for comfort and stability. It was a lesson reiterated as I transitioned into the corporate realm, where my commitment to transparency and truth collided with the harsh reality of organizational politics. It resonated deeply in the wake of personal loss when I was forced to confront the uncomfortable truth that life's journey is a perpetual series of changes.

Through these trials, I have come to understand that personal development is not about reaching a destination; it is about embracing the journey itself. It is about being willing to step into the unknown, even when it feels daunting, and to continually challenge myself to learn and grow. It is about recognizing that true growth often arises from moments of discomfort and vulnerability, as exemplified by my experiences navigating through unfamiliar territories and confronting the complexities of human relationships.

So, I have made a conscious choice not to shy away from life's challenges but to embrace them wholeheartedly. I have learned to view each obstacle as an opportunity for growth and each setback as a chance to deepen my understanding of myself and the world around me. In doing so, I have come to appreciate the beauty of life's ever-changing landscape, finding solace in the knowledge that, like the flow of the tide, personal growth is a constant, evolving journey.

6.4   Creating Your Guiding Principles

"Happiness is not a destination, it is a way of life."

Unknown - Source not attributed.

"Happiness is when what you think, what you say, and what you do are in harmony."

Mahatma Gandhi - India's independence movement leader

Objectives of the section

Build a set of principles or a personal code based on your identified values. This code will serve as a framework for decision-making and behaviors.

Key topics

DEFINE PERSONAL CODE - Develop a set of principles or guidelines based on your values.

CONSIDER EXTERNAL INFLUENCES - Be aware of external factors that may challenge your values. Understand how you want to respond to these challenges while maintaining your integrity and staying true to your principles.

REVIEW AND REVISE - Periodically review your principles and personal code. As you grow and evolve, your values may shift or become more refined. Adjust your personal code and principles accordingly.

Ray Dalio's journey to developing his approach to daily principles began early in his life. Raised in a middle-class family in Long Island, New York, Dalio exhibited a keen interest in the financial markets from a young age. Fascinated by the dynamics of the economy and the opportunities for wealth creation, he avidly studied investment strategies and market trends.

After graduating from Harvard Business School in 1973, Dalio founded Bridgewater Associates in his two-bedroom apartment in New York City. With a small team of dedicated colleagues, he began managing investments for clients, applying his unique approach to decision-making and risk management.

As Bridgewater Associates grew in size and reputation, Dalio encountered both success and challenges. He realized that traditional approaches to decision-making and leadership were insufficient for navigating the complexities of the financial markets and managing a rapidly expanding organization.

Determined to improve his effectiveness as a leader and investor, Dalio embarked on a journey of self-discovery and introspection. He spent years reflecting on his experiences, analyzing his successes and failures, and distilling the core principles that guided his decision-making.

Through this process of self-reflection and continuous learning, Dalio developed his approach to daily principles. Drawing inspiration from his own experiences and insights from psychology, economics, and philosophy, he articulated a set of principles that served as a foundation for his personal and professional life.

As Dalio implemented these principles within Bridgewater Associates, he witnessed profound transformations in the culture and performance of the organization. By fostering a culture of radical truth and transparency, encouraging systematic decision-making, and embracing reality as it is, Dalio and his team were able to navigate volatile markets, anticipate emerging trends, and achieve consistent success.

Today, Ray Dalio's approach to daily principles has become renowned worldwide, influencing countless individuals and organizations seeking to improve their decision-making processes and achieve greater success and fulfilment in life and work. Thus, his journey from a curious young investor to a visionary leader continues to inspire others to embrace the power of principles in their own lives. Here are three examples of some of the most impactful principles he uses:

Radical Truth and Transparency

This principle emphasizes the importance of fostering an environment where individuals feel comfortable sharing their thoughts, ideas, and feedback openly and honestly. By promoting radical truth and transparency, Dalio encourages constructive dialogue, effective problem-solving, and continuous learning within organizations. This principle enables teams to uncover hidden insights, address issues proactively, and make better-informed decisions.

Principle of "Pain + Reflection = Progress"

Dalio believes that embracing pain and failure as opportunities for reflection and learning is essential for personal and professional growth. This principle encourages individuals to confront their mistakes and setbacks head-on rather than avoiding or denying them. By reflecting on their experiences, identifying areas for improvement, and implementing changes, individuals can turn challenges into valuable learning opportunities and make meaningful progress towards their goals.

The Five-Step Process for Getting What You Want

This principle outlines a systematic approach to achieving desired outcomes in both personal and professional life. The five steps include setting clear goals, identifying and facing obstacles, diagnosing the root causes of problems, designing effective solutions, and implementing those solutions with discipline. By following this structured process, individuals can overcome obstacles, achieve their objectives, and continuously improve their performance over time.

These principles, among others, form the foundation of Ray Dalio's approach to decision-making and leadership, guiding individuals and organizations towards greater success and fulfilment.

In the turbulent waters of the 17th and 18th centuries, where ships sailed laden with treasure, and fear of pirates loomed large, a curious phenomenon emerged: the Pirates' Code. This was no ordinary set of rules; it was a testament to the democratic spirit that thrived amidst the lawless world of piracy.

Legend has it that beneath the tattered sails and weather-beaten decks of pirate ships, a form of governance emerged. Pirates, united by their desire for adventure and riches, found themselves in need of order amidst the chaos of the high seas. Thus, they convened in the dimly lit cabins and shadowy corners of their ships to draft their own laws - the Pirates' Code.

At the heart of this code lay the principle of equality. Regardless of one's background or station in life, each pirate was entitled to an equal share of the spoils acquired during their daring raids. This notion of equitable distribution fostered a sense of camaraderie among the crew, binding them together in their pursuit of fortune.

But the Pirates' Code went beyond mere division of loot; it embraced the ideals of democracy. Captains were not tyrants ruling with an iron fist but leaders chosen by the consent of the crew. Important decisions, whether it be selecting targets or electing leaders, were put to a vote, ensuring that every voice was heard and every opinion valued.

Yet, amidst the adventures and treasure hunts, the Pirates' Code also upheld principles of fairness and justice. Crew members were expected to treat one another with respect and dignity, and any transgressions were met with swift and decisive action.

In the perilous world of piracy, where danger lurked around every corner, the Pirates' Code served as a beacon of stability. It was a testament to the resilience and resourcefulness of those who sailed the seas in search of fortune and a reminder that even in the most lawless of lands, a semblance of order could be found. Some key principles of the Pirates' Code include:

Equal Distribution of Booty

Pirates believed in equitable sharing of plunder among crew members. According to the code, all spoils acquired during raids were to be divided fairly among the crew, with each member receiving an equal share based on their rank or contribution.

Democratic Decision-Making

Pirates operated under a democratic system of governance, where important decisions regarding the crew's activities, such as choosing targets or electing captains, were made collectively through a vote. This ensured that all crew members had a voice in the decision-making process.

Fair Treatment of Crew Members

The Pirates' Code emphasized the fair treatment of crew members and discouraged acts of cruelty or mistreatment. Captains were expected to uphold principles of fairness and justice in their dealings with the crew, and any violations of these principles could result in punishment or expulsion.

Mutual Protection and Support

Pirates recognized the importance of solidarity and mutual support among crew members. The code often included provisions for the protection of fellow pirates in times of danger, as well as rules governing disputes and conflicts within the crew.

Discipline and Order

Despite their reputation for lawlessness, pirates maintained a degree of discipline and order within their ranks. The code typically included rules and regulations governing conduct on board the ship, as well as penalties for disobedience or insubordination.

As the winds of change swept across the oceans and the era of piracy faded into legend, the legacy of the Pirates' Code endured. It stood as a testament to the spirit of those who dared to defy the norms of society and chart their own course amidst the vast expanse of the open sea.

Overall, the Pirates' Code reflected the unique social and cultural norms of pirate society, emphasizing principles of equality, democracy, and mutual cooperation among crew members. While pirates operated outside the boundaries of conventional law, their adherence to these codes helped maintain order and cohesion within their ranks during the Golden Age of Piracy.

Life principles and codes function as guiding frameworks, steering individuals towards meaningful and satisfying lives. They typically evolve from personal values, experiences, and beliefs, facilitating actions aligned with what matters most to us. These principles manifest uniquely in various contexts, whether applied to individuals or within relationships, be it romantic partnerships, familial dynamics, friendships, or professional settings.

The exploration of history is paramount to understanding who we are and what has brought us to where we are today. Delving into the historical principles that have shaped societal norms and laid the groundwork for contemporary ones is an intriguing endeavor.

Below, a condensed overview of various historical codes and their underlying principles is presented, spotlighting their central motivations and significance as drivers of societal evolution.

Guiding Moral Compass

The Ten Commandments uphold moral integrity, such as the prohibition against theft, fostering honesty and respect for property rights.

Virtuous Living

The Seven Virtues of Christianity cultivate qualities like patience and kindness, guiding individuals towards thoughtful and compassionate behavior.

Spiritual Duties and Charity

The Five Pillars of Islam outline fundamental religious obligations like prayer and charity, fostering community support and spiritual growth.

Path to Enlightenment

The Eightfold Path in Buddhism directs individuals towards enlightenment through mindful speech and compassionate actions, promoting harmony and understanding.

Justice and Fairness

The Code of Hammurabi establishes principles of justice, advocating for fair resolutions and proportional consequences in conflicts.

Ethical Conduct for Well-being

The Ten Precepts in Buddhism advocate ethical behavior, including compassion towards all living beings and environmental stewardship.

Embracing Truth and Balance

The Seven Principles of Maat from Ancient Egyptian philosophy prioritize truth and balance, guiding individuals towards integrity and harmony in life.

Code of Honor and Integrity

The Tenets of Bushido instill values like honor and loyalty, fostering personal integrity and responsibility even in challenging circumstances.

Prioritizing Harm Reduction

The Wiccan Rede emphasizes minimizing harm in decision-making, promoting thoughtful consideration of consequences for oneself and others.

Democratic Governance

The Pirate Code governs conduct among pirates, emphasizing democratic principles and fairness, ensuring equal treatment within pirate communities.

Utilizing these crucial historical codes and principles in their everyday experiences enables individuals to cultivate ethical behavior, mindfulness, and compassion in their conduct and interactions. This harmonization with personal values and life objectives enriches their sense of purpose and satisfaction.

Building upon these foundations and our accumulated insights over the years, we can organize a fundamental set of principles into ten distinct categories:

1. Integrity and honesty
2. Resilience and adaptability
3. Gratitude and positivity
4. Self-reflection and awareness
5. Empathy and compassion
6. Continuous learning and curiosity
7. Respecting and inclusivity
8. Balance and well-being
9. Purpose and meaning
10. Authenticity and genuine connections

The underlying principles and related codes for these key categories are further developed here under, supporting some practical examples applicable to determine actions in the case of individuals and various types of relationships. These can aid in your self-discovery journey and the formulation of your personal code.

Integrity and Honesty

Principle: Upholding moral and ethical standards.

Code: Being truthful and transparent in communication.

Examples

- Individual - Speaking truthfully, honoring commitments, and taking responsibility for one's actions.
- Relationships – Couples - Sharing thoughts and feelings openly with a partner, even when discussing difficult topics.
- Relationships - Friendship/Family - Keeping promises and commitments made to friends or family members.
- Work Interactions - Providing accurate information to colleagues, clients and suppliers, even when it may be challenging.

Resilience and Adaptability

Principle: Embracing challenges as opportunities for growth.

Code: Persisting in the face of adversity and adapting to changing circumstances.

Examples

- Individual - Learning from setbacks and using them as motivation to persevere and succeed.
- Relationships – Couples - Facing financial difficulties as a team and finding creative solutions together.
- Relationships - Friendship/Family - Being there for a friend going through a difficult breakup or loss.
- Work Interactions - Adjusting to new project requirements and working collaboratively to meet deadlines.

Gratitude and Positivity

Principle: Cultivating a positive outlook and expressing gratitude.

Code: Expressing appreciation for the good things in life.

Examples

- Individual - Starting each day with a gratitude journal or expressing thanks to loved ones.
- Relationships – Couples - Thanking a partner for their support and encouragement.
- Relationships - Friendship/Family - Acknowledging a friend's support during a challenging time.
- Work Interactions - Recognizing a coworker's efforts on a successful project.

Self-Reflection and Awareness

Principle: Regularly evaluating thoughts, actions, and motivations.

Code: Enhancing self-awareness through introspection.

Examples

- Individual - Setting aside time for introspection and journaling about personal experiences.

- Relationships – Couples - Reflecting on personal triggers and discussing them with a partner to deepen understanding.
- Relationships - Friendship/Family - Recognizing personal biases and actively listening to others' perspectives during a family discussion.
- Work Interactions - Seeking feedback from supervisors and peers to identify opportunities for growth.

Empathy and Compassion

Principle: Seeking to understand and share the feelings of others.

Code: Showing kindness and consideration.

Examples

- Individual - Listening empathetically to a friend going through a tough time and offering support.
- Relationships – Couples - Showing empathy towards a partner's feelings and offering comfort during times of stress.
- Relationships - Friendship/Family - Providing a shoulder to lean on and offering practical help to a family member facing challenges.
- Work Interactions - Acknowledging a coworker's workload and offering assistance or support.

Continuous Learning and Curiosity

Principle: Embracing a mindset of lifelong learning.

Code: Seeking out new experiences and knowledge.

Examples

- Individual - Taking up a new hobby or enrolling in an online course to expand knowledge and skills.
- Relationships – Couples - Trying out new activities together and sharing insights gained from personal interests.
- Relationships - Friendship/Family - Discussing books, movies, or current events with friends or family members to exchange perspectives.

- Work Interactions - Attending industry conferences or workshops to stay updated on best practices and trends.

Respecting and Inclusivity

Principle: Treating others with dignity and consideration.

Code: Valuing diversity and different perspectives.

Examples

- Individual - Listening respectfully to someone with opposing views and engaging in constructive dialogue.
- Relationships – Couples - Respecting a partner's boundaries and opinions, even if they differ from one's own.
- Relationships - Friendship/Family - Celebrating cultural traditions and respecting personal beliefs within the family or friend group.
- Work Interactions - Seeking input from team members with diverse backgrounds and experiences during decision-making processes.

Balance and Well-being

Principle: Prioritizing balance in various aspects of life.

Code: Supporting personal health and wellness.

Examples

- Individual - Setting boundaries on work hours and making time for leisure activities or self-care practices.
- Relationships – Couples - Encouraging a partner to take breaks and pursue hobbies outside of work to reduce stress.
- Relationships - Friendship/Family - Planning family outings or gatherings that accommodate everyone's schedules and interests.
- Work Interactions - Offering flexible work arrangements or wellness programs to support employees' physical and mental health.

Purpose and Meaning

Principle: Defining and pursuing life's purpose or meaning.

Code: Aligning actions with personal values and long-term goals.

Examples

- Individual - Setting specific goals related to career advancement, personal development, or contributions to society.
- Relationships – Couples - Discussing future plans and aspirations as a couple and supporting each other's individual goals.
- Relationships - Friendship/Family - Volunteering together for a charitable cause or supporting a family member's educational pursuits.
- Work Interactions - Communicating how each team member's contributions participate in the company's overall success and impact.

Authenticity and Genuine Connections

Principle: Building trust and rapport through authenticity.

Code: Being true to oneself and fostering genuine connections.

Examples

- Individual - Sharing personal experiences and vulnerabilities authentically to deepen relationships.
- Relationships – Couples - Having honest conversations about fears or insecurities with a partner and being receptive to their feedback and support.
- Relationships - Friendship/Family - Being supportive and non-judgmental when a friend or family member shares their struggles or challenges.
- Work Interactions - Encouraging open dialogue and feedback during team meetings or brainstorming sessions, allowing everyone to contribute ideas without fear of judgment.

By applying these principles and codes in their daily lives, individuals can cultivate meaningful relationships, promote personal growth, and contribute positively to their communities and workplaces.

Remember that developing life principles and a personal code is an ongoing process. It requires self-awareness, introspection, and a commitment to living in accordance with your values. Adjustment may be necessary as life circumstances change, but having a solid foundation will help you navigate challenges and stay true to yourself.

6.4.1 Defining your personal code and principles

Here are steps to help you define your life principles and craft a personal code that aligns with your values:

1. Define Your Personal Code: Establish a set of principles or guidelines based on your values. This may involve committing to honesty, kindness, continuous learning, or other qualities that deeply resonate with you.
2. Consider External Influences: Stay mindful of external factors that might test your values. Determine how you wish to respond to these influences while upholding your integrity and remaining faithful to your principles.
3. Review and Revise: Regularly assess your principles and personal code. As you undergo growth and development, your values may evolve or become more refined. Adjust your personal code accordingly to reflect these changes.

My personal code and principles

While formulating my personal principles, I focused on the values outlined in Section 6.3.1, specifically:

- Justice and fairness
- Respect
- Trust
- Personal development and challenges

Drawing connections with the principles outlined in this section, I correlated my values with the following:

- *Respecting and inclusivity*: This involves treating others with dignity and consideration, embracing diversity, and valuing different perspectives, which inherently includes ensuring respect as well as justice and fairness for all.
- *Integrity and honesty*: These principles form the foundation of trust.
- *Self-reflection and awareness*: This serves as the cornerstone of personal growth, fostering awareness of one's strengths, weaknesses, and areas for improvement.
- *Purpose and meaning*: This complements the values of trust, justice and fairness by emphasizing the importance of aligning actions with long-term goals and dreams, fostering authentic connections based on shared values.

Additionally, I incorporated a recently emphasized principle in my life: "Balance and well-being," as I have been focusing more on consistent exercise and dietary adjustments. From these considerations, my personal principles translate into the following:

Integrity and honesty

- Foster trust and openness in relationships by consistently sharing important information.
- Express emotions, even if uncomfortable.
- Seek clarification when principles are unclear, acknowledging that adherence is not always automatic.

Self-reflection and awareness / Continuous learning and curiosity

- Embrace the evolving nature of each day's behaviors.
- Avoid setting default limits for myself or others.

Respecting and inclusivity

- Avoid imposing pressure or obligations on myself or others, prioritizing understanding and empathy.
- Refrain from judgment and instead seek to understand others' emotions and perspectives.

Balance and well-being

- Maintain a consistent balance between physical, psychological, and spiritual health, adhering to a structured workout plan and daily reading regimen.

Purpose and meaning

- Consistently align actions with long-term objectives and dreams, following the process of "The Gray Spot."

6.5 Dream Exploration: Unveiling Your Deepest Desires

"If you want to be happy, set a goal that commands your thoughts, liberates your energy, and inspires your hopes."

Andrew Carnegie - Scottish-American industrialist and philanthropist.

"The purpose of our lives is to be happy."

Dalai Lama XIV - Tibetan spiritual leader

Objectives of the section

Explore your personal dreams and wishes - Uncover your deepest desires and aspirations and delve into them to identify your deepest dreams and wishes. Leverage them to shape life's direction.

Key topics

IDENTIFY YOUR DREAMS AND WISHES – Clarify your dreams and wishes, rooted in genuine passion and purpose and aligned with your authentic self. These should be aligned with your key values,

DETERMINE CLEAR GOALS – Translate your dreams and wishes into life goals in alignment with your principles.

REFLECTION - Reflect on what truly matters to you and what you would crave to accomplish if there were no external influences from the environment, others, and societal expectations.

The Montgomery Bus Boycott, sparked by Rosa Parks in 1955, gained momentum as Martin Luther King Jr. emerged as a charismatic leader. Pivotal moments included the formation of the Montgomery Improvement Association (MIA), led by King, which orchestrated the boycott. The unity within the black community, sustained over 381 days of walking instead of using buses, showcased a shared commitment to change.

The success was driven by nonviolent resistance, exemplified by the Montgomery Bus Boycott, which drew national attention. Legal battles declaring bus segregation unconstitutional underscored the movement's achievements. The boycott highlighted the power of organized activism, leveraging networks to amplify the message, and instilled a legacy of civil rights activism.

Personal values and life dreams played a crucial role in the success of the Montgomery Bus Boycott. Rosa Parks' strong conviction in her personal value of dignity fueled her refusal to give up her bus seat, setting the stage for the movement. Martin Luther King Jr.'s dream of racial equality and justice became a driving force, uniting individuals with a shared vision.

The commitment of countless participants reflected their deeply held values of equality and fairness. The boycott demonstrated how aligning personal values with a collective dream could mobilize a community. It showcased that when individuals passionately pursue dreams rooted in justice, it can lead to transformative social change, emphasizing the profound impact of personal values on the broader pursuit of civil rights.

Rooted in Rosa Parks' refusal and fueled by Martin Luther King Jr.'s dream, the Montgomery Bus Boycott epitomized the fusion of personal values and collective vision. Through 381 days of walking, legal battles, and the formation of the MIA, individuals showcased an unyielding commitment to justice. This historic movement underscored how personal values, like Parks' dignity and dreams of equality, as embodied by King, could ignite transformative change, leaving an indelible mark on the fight for civil rights.

During my childhood, I was always captivated by the prospect of crafting my Christmas wish list or pondering about my future career aspirations when prompted by my primary school teachers. These moments sparked a flurry of excitement as I envisioned a world without constraints, where my deepest desires could manifest freely.

However, this utopian vision often collided with the harshness of reality, ushering in a sobering dose of pragmatism. The innocent wish for an excavator under the Christmas tree was gently redirected by my parents to a more feasible alternative—a Lego model. Similarly, my lofty ambition of becoming an astronaut was met with the stern guidance of a professional counselor, who emphasized the importance of laying down a solid foundation in mathematics and physics before venturing into the cosmos.

These encounters with reality served as pivotal moments where the exuberance of youthful dreams met the tempered wisdom of practicality. While my aspirations may have been initially trimmed to fit within the bounds of plausibility, they also instilled in me a resilience and adaptability that would prove invaluable in navigating the complexities of adulthood.

When we contemplate life's journey from the vantage point of our final moments, what memories do we cherish? As loved ones gather by our bedside, inquiring about our deepest regrets, how do we envision our responses? The longing to depart without lingering remorse is a universal aspiration, yet one seldom fully realized. For many, regrets originate from yielding to external influences—societal norms, environmental pressures, and circumstantial constraints dictating our choices.

Common regrets resonate with the echoes of unspoken emotions, missed opportunities for connection, and forsaken personal passions. The sorrow of inadequate time spent nurturing relationships or failing to prioritize what truly matters reverberates deeply within us. Regrets, classified into distinct domains, leave indelible marks on our lives, shaping our trajectories and informing our future decisions. These domains include:

Personal Integrity - Serving as a cornerstone, regrets arise from compromising values or failing to advocate for oneself or others.

Relationships - Essential to the human experience, regrets stem from neglecting significant relationships, insufficient time spent with loved ones, unexpressed emotions, or unresolved conflicts.

Work-Life Balance - Reflects regrets born from the relentless pursuit of a career, financial gain, and status at the expense of personal fulfilment.

Health and Self-Care - Often overlooked amid other pursuits, regrets intertwine with well-being, reflecting neglect or underestimation of its importance.

Personal Development - Reveals remorse over forsaken aspirations, neglected passions, or hesitations to pursue dreams.

Contemplating these regrets underscores the significance of aligning our life choices with personal objectives—a guiding North Star illuminating the path towards fulfilment. Dreams and wishes, embodiments of our deepest desires and aspirations, infuse vitality into life's journey, serving as beacons of purpose and propelling us toward growth and self-discovery.

Yet, while dreaming is essential, navigating the chasm between aspiration and reality demands a delicate balance. Society's inclination to confine individuals within rigid frameworks stifles creativity and inhibits innovation. Conformity, reinforced by standardized systems and societal expectations, often obstructs the pursuit of authentic passions.

Being dreamful can indeed ignite the fires of ambition; lacking a connection to reality can lead to venturing into dangerous territory. Blindly chasing dreams without assessing the present landscape can lead to disillusionment and squandered opportunities. However, initiating the process of defining personal dreams and wishes, unshackled by limitations, is crucial for individual growth and development. By articulating our aspirations, we gain clarity on our motivations, paving the way for strategic actions toward personal fulfilment.

My childhood experiences can serve as an illustration of the clash between youthful dreams and the harsh realities of societal norms. The pressure to conform often stifles innovation and suppresses grand ambitions, confining individuals to predefined boxes. This limitation not only impedes personal growth but also obstructs the pursuit of happiness. Society's imposition of rigid educational systems and societal expectations exacerbates this issue, stifling creativity and diverting individuals from their true passions.

Moreover, individuals grapple with internal barriers—self-doubt, fear of failure, and reluctance to step beyond comfort zones—that restrain their potential. Overcoming these constraints requires resilience, a growth mindset, and environments conducive to risk-taking and creativity. Bridging the chasm between aspiration and reality necessitates grounding lofty dreams in pragmatic steps, fostering adaptability and resourcefulness along the journey.

Balancing boundless dreams with pragmatic reality entails charting a realistic path toward those aspirations. This involves setting achievable short-term goals aligned with broader dreams while acknowledging and working within existing limitations. Adaptability and resourcefulness are vital, enabling individuals to pivot their approach as needed while staying rooted in practical steps toward their dreams.

In navigating the complexities of modern society, effective communication, empathy, and a willingness to embrace diverse perspectives are essential. Seeking common ground and fostering dialogue facilitate the discovery of shared goals, leading to collaborative solutions benefiting all parties involved. Flexibility and a collaborative mindset are indispensable in transcending rigid viewpoints, nurturing inclusivity, and fostering harmony in society.

To effectively uncover your life dreams and desires, it is crucial to intertwine your aspirations with your core values, inherent talents, and acquired skills. This holistic approach not only fosters happiness but also enhances the feasibility of realizing your dreams based on your current state and self-awareness. Segmenting your aspirations into categories aids in maintaining a well-rounded personal development strategy that aligns with your values and long-term vision.

These categories may encompass (but are not limited to):

- *Career*: Objectives related to professional advancement, such as career milestones and pursuing a specific vocational path.
- *Personal Development*: Goals for self-improvement encompassing education, self-awareness, and emotional intelligence.
- *Relationship*: Dreams centered around meaningful connections with family, friends, and partners.
- *Health*: Ambitions for physical and mental well-being, including fitness, nutrition, and overall lifestyle choices.
- *Hobbies*: Activities that bring joy and fulfilment outside of work, contributing to personal satisfaction.
- *Financial Goals*: Aspirations regarding savings, investments, and achieving financial stability.
- *Travel*: Desires to explore new places and cultures, creating lasting memories.
- *Contribution to Others*: Aspirations for making a positive impact on the community or world through volunteering or charitable work.

- *Learning*: Goals for continuous intellectual growth and skill acquisition.
- *Spiritual Growth*: Aspirations for inner peace and a deeper connection with spirituality or beliefs.

And are represented visually on the cards here:

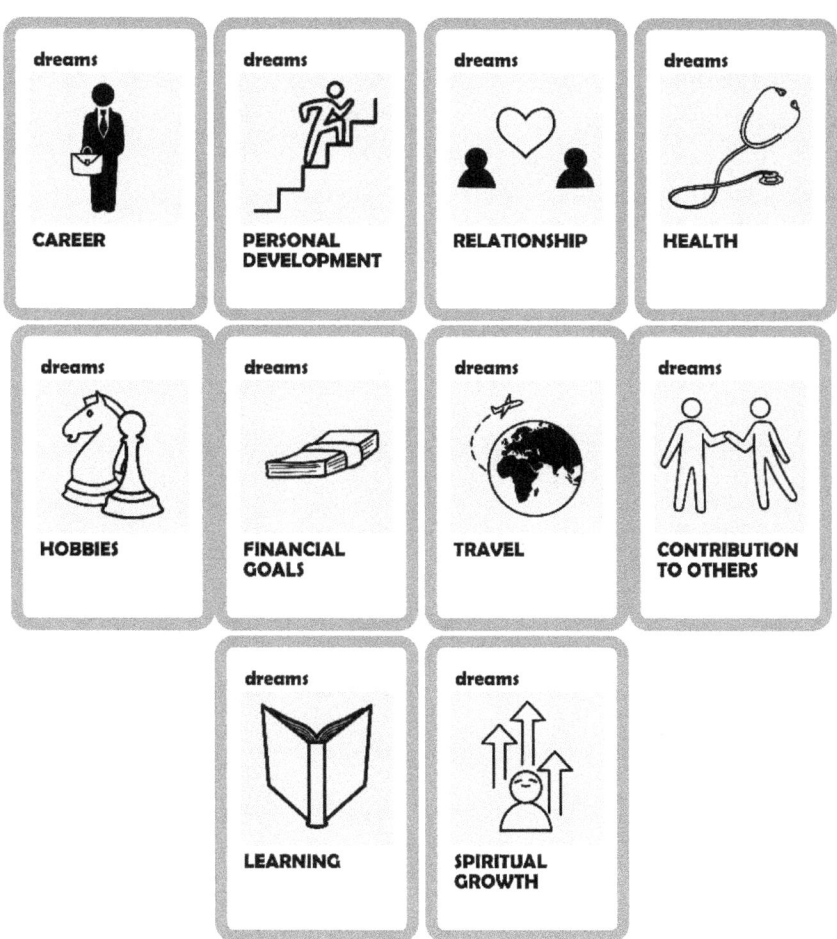

After identifying your dreams, it is essential to assess your confidence in their ability to bring happiness and their realism based on your capabilities and gifts. Visualization techniques, such as the following ones, can aid in this process:

- Create Vivid Mental Pictures - Imagine your goals with clarity, engaging all your senses to evoke the emotions associated with achieving them.
- Visualize Daily - Dedicate regular time to envisioning your dreams, strengthening neural connections, and reinforcing belief in their attainability.
- Positive Affirmations - Combine affirmations with visualizations to boost self-belief and confidence.

Supplemental techniques such as dream journals, lucid dreaming, visualization exercises, and external stimuli can further enhance your dream exploration. These methods offer unique advantages and considerations, emphasizing individual preferences and goals.

6.5.1 Determine your personal dreams and wishes

As discussed here above, a strategic approach to identifying your life objectives begins with clarifying your dreams and wishes. By delving into your past experiences and values, you can envision your aspirations for the future with greater depth. Here are some key steps to guide you through this process:

1. Take time to reflect on the life you envision for yourself and the legacy you aim to leave behind. Engaging in introspection and reflection empowers you to articulate your personal meaning in life, laying the groundwork for living authentically and with purpose. To aid this process, you can utilize the significant events identified in Section 6.2 and visualize them through the cards you selected.

2. Consider any regrets you might have if you were to leave this world today. Reflecting on these regrets can provide valuable insights into your deepest desires and priorities.

3. Categorize your future dreams and wishes into distinct areas. This segmentation helps organize your thoughts and allows for a clearer understanding of your aspirations across different aspects of life.

4. Evaluate the confidence and realism of your defined dreams, considering your personal skills, gifts, and external factors. Additionally, weigh the balance between expected happiness and potential discomfort, the risks involved versus stability, and the degree of freedom versus reliance on external factors.

By consistently engaging in this process, you embark on a journey of self-discovery that transforms your understanding of identity, values, and aspirations. This transformative exploration illuminates the path toward personal fulfilment, guiding you toward a life aligned with your deepest desires.

My personal dreams and wishes

Upon reflecting on the first forty-five years of my life, I came to realize that my environment had exerted a strong influence on me, and I had never taken the time to contemplate my aspirations until much later in life. Beginning my journey of self-discovery, I started to ponder what I truly wished to accomplish and began compiling a list of tangible actions. These aspirations ranged from becoming a certified Scuba diver and writing a book to learning to play the drums and establishing a rock band, improving my fitness, creating a company, and dedicating quality time to my family, among others.

While these pursuits were instrumental in my personal development and fulfilment, I recognized an absence of a higher-level sense of purpose, akin to a guiding North Star, to steer me toward actions that would propel me forward.

Investing additional time in understanding my key motivators and what would bring satisfaction to my life, I expanded upon this by identifying the paramount categories and defining my guiding aspirations. These include:

Thriving in a career with meaningful connections

Categories: Career / Relationship

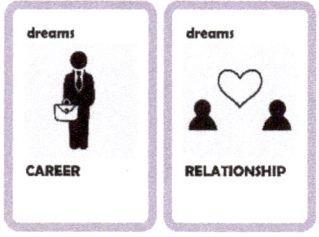

Aspiration: Cultivating a fulfilling career aligned with my passions while fostering meaningful connections with like-minded individuals.

Experiencing unconditional love in a fulfilling relationship

Categories: Relationship / Contribution to others

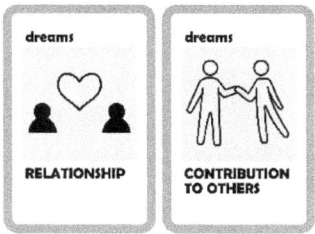

Aspiration: Pursuing a loving and unrestricted relationship, prioritizing compatibility and open communication to establish a deep connection.

Achieving a comfortable, balanced life free from external pressures

Categories: Financial Goals / Health / Relationship

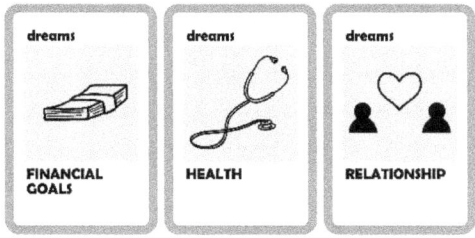

Aspiration: Striving for a comfortable, balanced life by managing finances wisely, prioritizing self-care, and establishing healthy boundaries in both personal and professional relationships.

Pursuing continuous development through a balanced spectrum of activities

Categories: Personal Development / Learning / Hobbies / Health

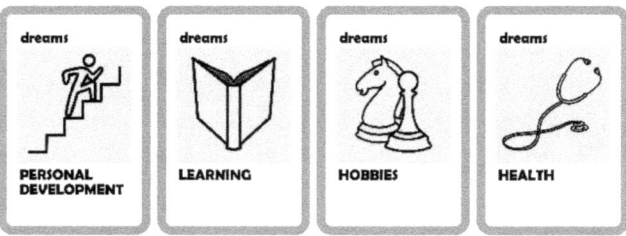

Aspiration: Engaging in a variety of challenging activities that stimulate physical, emotional, and spiritual growth on a continuous basis.

6.6   Set practical objectives and related actions

"Happiness is not something ready-made. It comes from your own actions."

Dalai Lama XIV – Tibetan spiritual leader

Objectives of the section

Take intentional and consistent actions to achieve your goals. Your personal code and values should guide your actions, helping you stay on course and navigate challenges with integrity.

Key topics

SET CLEAR GOALS – Establish short-term and long-term goals aligned with your dreams and wishes. Your life principles should guide you towards achieving these goals in a way that stays true to your values.

INTEGRATE INTO DAILY LIFE – Actively apply your principles in your daily life. Consider how your values guide your decisions, relationships, and actions. Address common obstacles that may hinder goal pursuit.

LEARN FROM MISTAKES – Embrace the learning opportunities that come from mistakes. Use them to refine your principles and reinforce your commitment to your values.

SHARE AND DIALOGUE – Communicate your principles with those close to you. Engage in dialogues about values and learn from others. This can provide valuable insights and strengthen your commitment to your personal code.

Building upon the established principles, actions can be meticulously crafted, drawing upon personal values, principles, and past experiences to propel you toward the realization of your personal aspirations, dreams, and desires. These actions should resonate deeply with your core values, guiding principles, and the lessons gleaned from your own journey. In addition, for optimum effectiveness, these actions should adhere to the SMART criteria, which is an acronym standing for:

- *Specific*: Goals should be clear and well-defined. They should answer the questions: What do I want to accomplish? Why is this goal important? Who is involved? Where is it located? What resources or limits are involved?
- *Measurable*: Goals should be quantifiable. It should be possible to track progress and determine when the goal has been achieved. Ask questions like: How much? How many? How will I know when it is accomplished?
- *Achievable*: Goals should be realistic and attainable. They should stretch your abilities but still remain possible to achieve. It is important to consider whether the goal is within your control and whether you have the necessary resources and capabilities to accomplish it.
- *Relevant*: Goals should align with your broader objectives and be meaningful to you and the people you interact with. They should contribute to your overall mission and vision. Ask yourself: Does this goal matter? Is it worthwhile? Is now the right time?
- *Time-bound*: Goals should have a deadline or target date. This creates a sense of urgency and helps prevent procrastination. It is essential to set a timeframe for achieving the goal. Ask: When will I work on this? What can I do six months from now? What can I do six weeks from now? What can I do today?

To be truly effective, each action should embody a deep understanding of personal values, serving as a manifestation of what truly matters. Anchoring actions in personal ethos ensures each step is meaningful, contributing authentically to success and fulfilment. Integrating principles from past experiences enhances action efficacy, leveraging insights from successes and setbacks to refine approaches.

When defining actions, it is crucial to consider not only what needs doing but also why it matters personally. Actions should reflect purpose rooted in values and principles, ensuring alignment between objectives and authentic selves. Action definitions are not just task outlines but deliberate integrations of personal values, principles, and experiences into the journey towards dreams and aspirations.

Actions should start with a verb, embody a distinct theme, include a quantifiable gauge of success, and have a timeline for accomplishment. Objectives should harmonize with aspirations, values, and reflections on what holds significance. Differentiating between internal motivators and external influences is key, achieved through regular introspection to maintain alignment with authentic selves. A repertoire of potential actions may include:

- Learn
- Reflect
- Grow
- Adapt
- Improve
- Develop
- Challenge
- Transform
- Achieve
- Evolve

You will find here some representations on related cards:

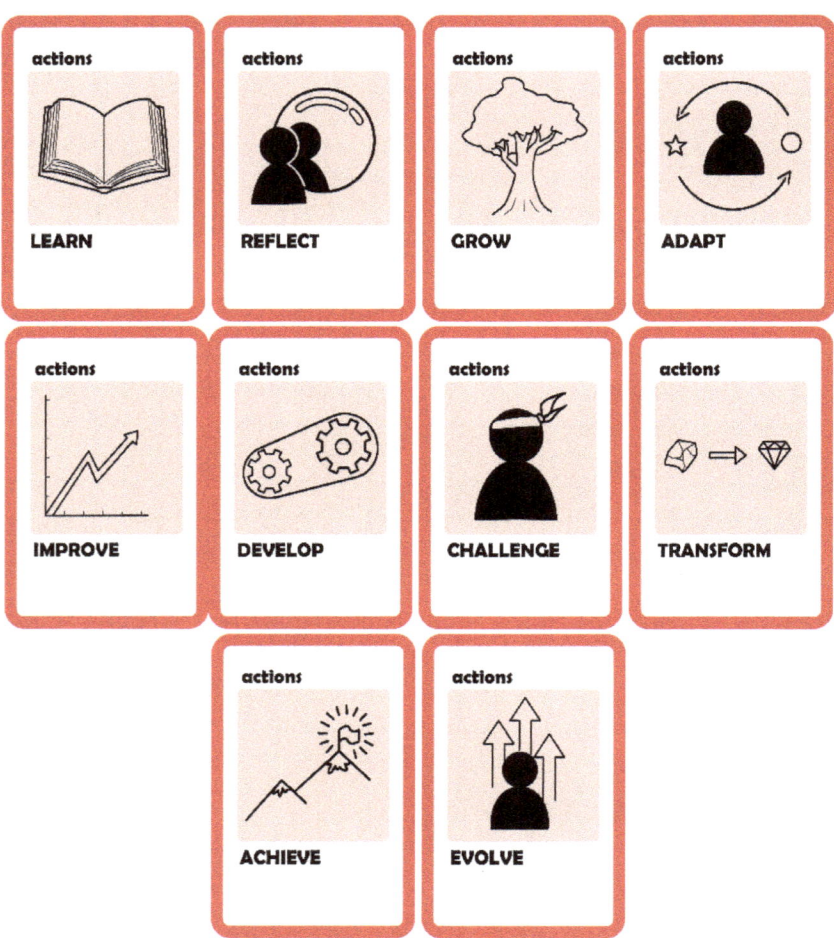

During reflection on pivotal events, values, principles, and identified dreams, determine actions for the coming weeks and months. Write them down with action verbs, tie them to environments and relationships, anticipate emotions upon realization, and match them with related cards.

6.6.1 Determine your personal goals and actions.

To fulfil your personal aspirations, dreams, and desires, it is crucial to outline and implement key actions that propel you toward your personal guiding light. This requires following a consistent and structured approach. Here is a proposed method:

1. Reflect on your dreams, wishes, and aspirations (leveraging on Section 6.5).
2. Assess your current situation to identify what is needed to bridge the potential gaps (leveraging on Section 6.2).
3. Ensure alignment with your values and principles (leveraging on Sections 6.3 and 6.4) to authentically connect your dreams with your true self before delineating concrete actions.
4. Define three to five short- and mid-term actions that will bring you closer to realizing your dreams, ensuring they adhere to the SMART concept and instill confidence in execution.
5. Incorporate the context, individuals involved, and anticipated emotions into the defined actions.
6. Continuously revisit the process as actions are completed or life circumstances evolve, making necessary adjustments along the way.

As previously mentioned, you can leverage the cards describing the defining aspects of your personal self to support a more efficient visualization.

Upon reflection on the aspirations that I outlined in Section 6.5.1, my following key desires for life emerged:

- *Thriving in a career with meaningful connections* - Cultivating a fulfilling career aligned with my passions while fostering meaningful connections with like-minded individuals
- *Experiencing unconditional love in a fulfilling relationship* - Pursuing a loving and unrestricted relationship, prioritizing compatibility, and open communication to establish a deep connection.
- *Achieving a comfortable, balanced life free from external pressures* - Striving for a comfortable, balanced life by managing finances wisely, prioritizing self-care, and establishing healthy boundaries in both personal and professional relationships.
- *Pursuing continuous development through a balanced spectrum of activities* - Engaging in a variety of challenging activities that stimulate physical, emotional, and spiritual growth on a continuous basis.

Recognizing these aspirations, I have pinpointed critical gaps impeding progress towards fulfilling my life goals:

Thriving in a career with meaningful connections:

- Limited networking beyond immediate professional needs despite active involvement in my field.
- Lack of alignment between my job and personal values resulted in a lack of passion in daily interactions.

Experiencing unconditional love in a fulfilling relationship:

- Despite an outwardly peaceful family life, I struggled to express thoughts and feelings openly, feeling constrained by external influences akin to experiences from childhood.

Achieving a comfortable, balanced life free from external pressures:

- Financial success in my career juxtaposed with blurred boundaries between personal and professional life, thus presenting challenges.

Pursuing continuous development through a balanced spectrum of activities:

- I neglected personal growth while focusing on work and family responsibilities, leading to imbalance and potential instability.

By connecting them back with my key principles derived in Section 6.4.1 in close alignment with my personal values, namely:

Integrity and honesty

- Foster trust and openness in relationships by consistently sharing important information.
- Express emotions, even if uncomfortable.
- Seek clarification when principles are unclear, acknowledging that adherence is not always automatic.

Self-reflection and awareness / Continuous learning and curiosity

- Embrace the evolving nature of each day's behaviors.
- Avoid setting default limits for myself or others.

Respecting and inclusivity

- Avoid imposing pressure or obligations on myself or others, prioritizing understanding, and empathy.
- Refrain from judgment and instead seek to understand others' emotions and perspectives.

Balance and well-being

- Maintain a consistent balance between physical, psychological, and spiritual health, adhering to a structured workout plan and daily reading regimen.

Purpose and meaning

- Consistently align actions with long-term objectives and dreams, following the process of "The Gray Spot."

I have consolidated actionable steps and derived subsequent short- and mid-term actions. Addressing these gaps necessitates establishing a balanced and sustainable framework of priorities, as will be detailed in Section 7.1, which introduces the concept of life-supporting pillars.

ACTION 1 - Growing, Developing, Challenging, Achieving

Dream / wish: Thriving in a career with meaningful connections.

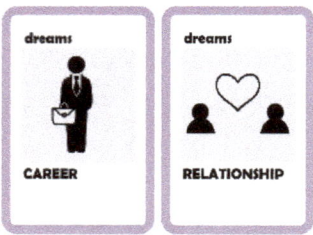

Principle: Integrity and honesty / Purpose and meaning

Action: Enhance my network by cultivating authentic relationships with individuals who resonate with my values and goals, supporting them in their endeavors while also seeking avenues for career growth within this network. I have committed to creating or maintaining at least three such connections each week.

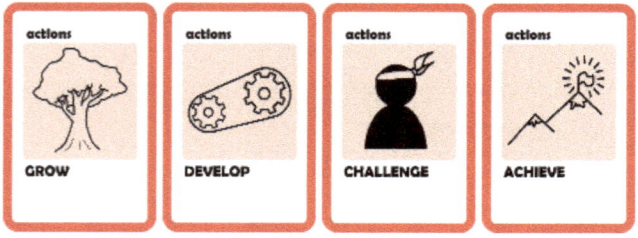

Environment: Workplace / Social events

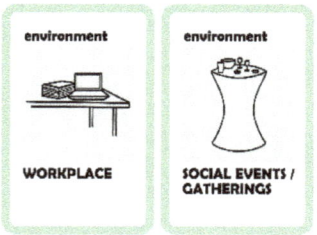

Relationship: Colleagues / Friends

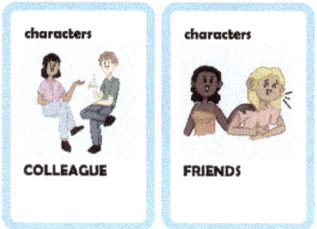

Expected positive emotions: Gratitude / Pride / Confidence

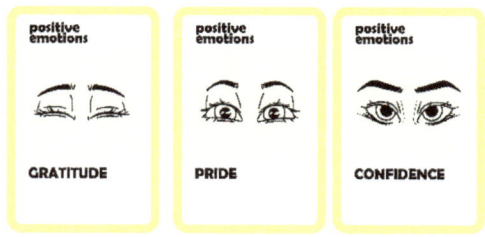

ACTION 2 - Reflecting, Growing, Achieving, Transforming

Dream/wish: Experiencing unconditional love in a fulfilling relationship.

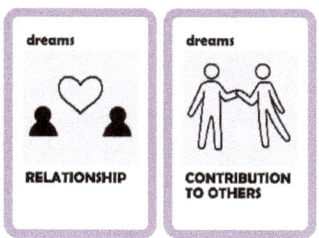

Principle: Integrity and honesty / Respecting and inclusivity

Action: Promote openness and authenticity through regular and structured communication of thoughts and emotions, actively engaging in discussions about emotional well-being with loved ones. A strategy I have implemented to facilitate this is consistently asking and answering the following questions during interactions with my partner: "How are you/am I doing with yourself/myself? How are you/am I doing with me/you? How are you/am I doing with others?

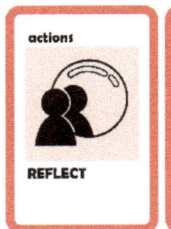 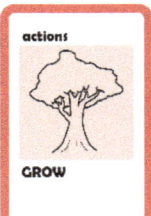 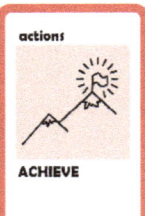 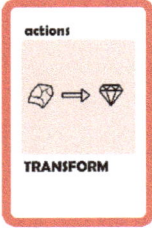

Environment: Home

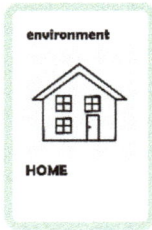

Relationship: Partner

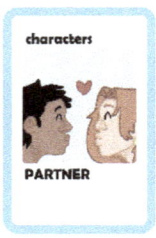

Expected positive emotions: Love / Serenity / Confidence

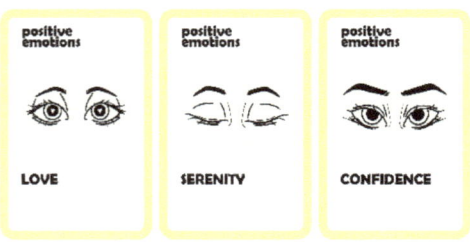

ACTION 3 - Adapting, Developing, Improving, Achieving

Dream/wish: Achieving a comfortable, balanced life free from external pressures.

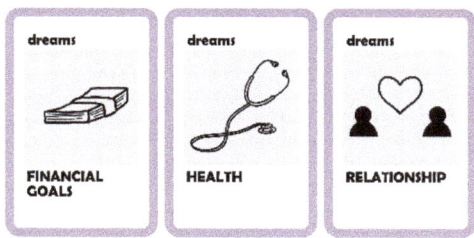

Principle: Balance and well-being

Action: Set distinct boundaries in both personal and professional domains, placing emphasis on self-care and mental wellness by allocating specific time for physical, mental, and spiritual practices. Specifically, I've implemented the following routines:

- Engaging in a one-hour workout six times a week
- Devoting at least 30 minutes daily to reading material that prompts personal reflection and contemplation
- Allocating at least two half-days each month for leisure pursuits like drum playing, songwriting, or scuba diving

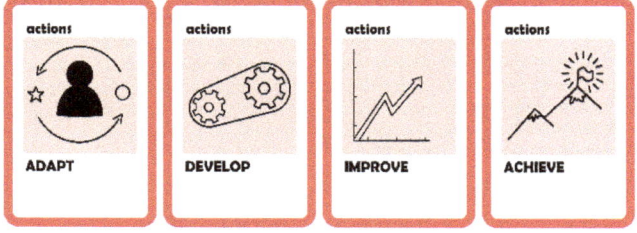

Environment: Home / Workplace

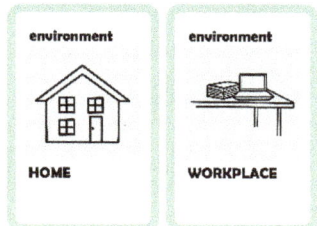

Relationship: Partner / Friends / Children

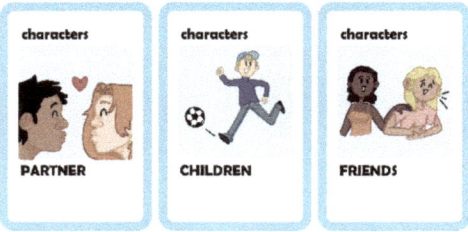

Expected positive emotions: Gratitude / Contentment

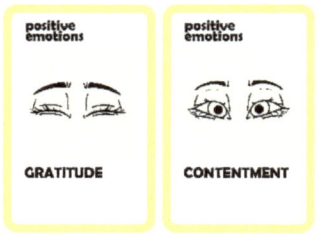

ACTION 4 – Learning, Reflecting, Growing, Adapting, Improving, Developing, Achieving

Dream/wish: Pursuing continuous development through a balanced spectrum of activities.

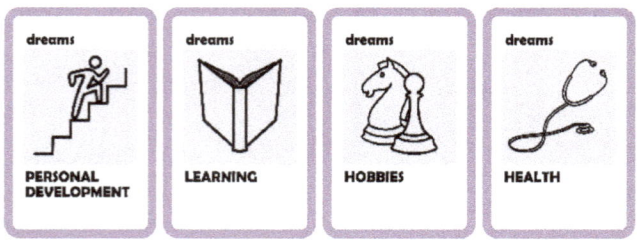

Principle: Self-reflection and awareness / Continuous learning and curiosity / Purpose and meaning

Action: Evaluate performance on priorities every three months, adjusting to maintain alignment with values and "The Gray Spot" approach.

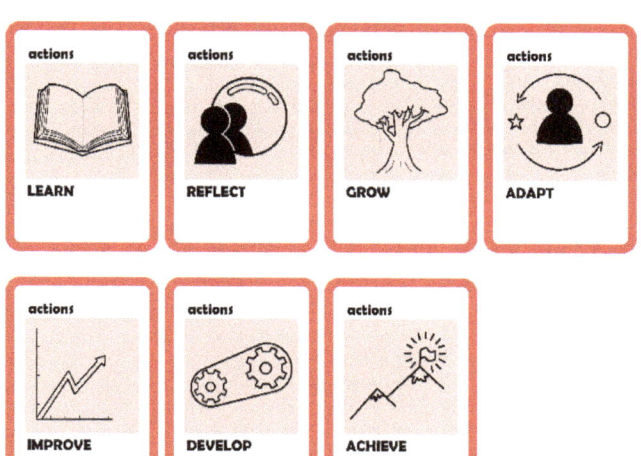

Environment: Home / Workplace / Outdoor spaces / Social gatherings

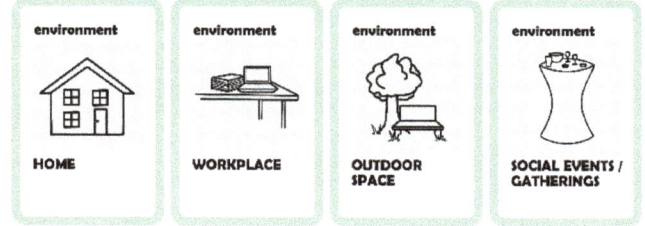

Relationship: Friends/Hobby mates/Alone

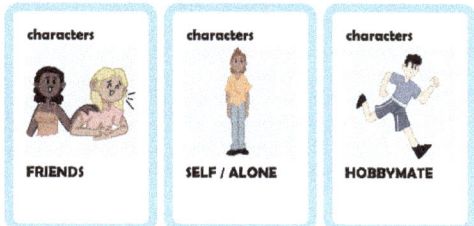

Expected emotions: Joy/Contentment / Excitement / Inspiration

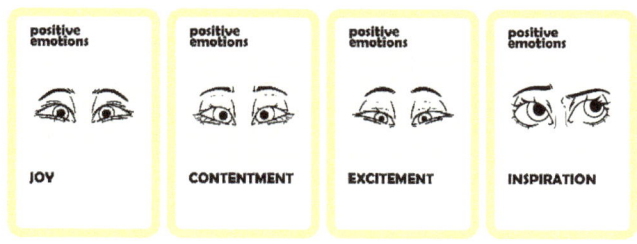

7 "The Gray Spot" model

"Happiness is not the absence of problems, it is the ability to deal with them."

Steve Maraboli - Behavioral scientist, author

"Happiness is a choice, not a result. Nothing will make you happy until you choose to be happy."

Ralph Marston - Motivational writer and publisher.

One poignant example illustrating the evolution from individual identity to integration within a societal system is the remarkable journey of Nelson Mandela. His narrative vividly portrays the intricate interplay of self-awareness, personal values and beliefs, principles, life objectives, and the actions undertaken to realize dreams and achieve goals.

Nelson Mandela embarked on his journey with a profound understanding of his identity, deeply rooted in his Xhosa heritage and upbringing in South Africa. From an early age, he was imbued with a strong sense of self-awareness, recognizing his place within his community and the broader societal context.

Driven by his unwavering personal values and beliefs, Mandela was compelled to confront the injustices perpetuated by the apartheid regime. His core principles of justice, equality, and freedom were the guiding forces that propelled him into the arena of political activism.

With a clear vision of his life objectives and dreams for a liberated South Africa, Mandela fearlessly embarked on a path of resistance against oppression. Despite facing numerous obstacles and risks, which let him endure decades of imprisonment, persecution, and personal sacrifice in the pursuit of freedom and equality for all South Africans, he remained steadfast in his commitment to realizing his aspirations for a just and equitable society.

Mandela's actions were characterized by courage, resilience, and strategic foresight. He engaged in a range of activities, from grassroots organizing to international diplomacy, all aimed at fulfilling his dreams and achieving his goals of ending apartheid and establishing democracy.

Throughout his journey, Mandela's personal principles served as a moral compass, guiding his decisions and actions even in the face of adversity. His unwavering commitment to non-violence and reconciliation became emblematic of his leadership style and contributed to his ability to unite diverse factions within South African society.

In essence, Nelson Mandela's story exemplifies the intricate interplay between self-awareness, personal values, principles, life objectives, and actions in the pursuit of societal transformation. His journey serves as a testament to the power of individual agency and collective action in effecting positive change and shaping the course of history.

An example of a journey where the evolution from individual identity to integration within a societal system was ultimately unsuccessful is that of Socrates, the ancient Greek philosopher.

Socrates was a figure deeply rooted in self-awareness, possessing a profound understanding of his identity as a philosopher and a citizen of Athens. He dedicated his life to the pursuit of knowledge, guided by personal values and beliefs centered on truth, virtue, and the examination of one's own life.

Driven by his principles, Socrates sought to challenge the conventions and norms of Athenian society through his philosophical inquiries. He engaged in dialogue with fellow citizens, questioning their assumptions and beliefs, often leading to discomfort and resistance among the Athenian elite.

Socrates' life objectives and dreams were focused on fostering intellectual enlightenment and moral improvement within Athenian society. He believed that by encouraging critical thinking and self-reflection, he could contribute to the betterment of individuals and the collective community.

However, despite his noble intentions and tireless efforts, Socrates' actions ultimately led to his downfall. His relentless questioning of authority and his refusal to compromise his principles brought him into conflict with the ruling elite of Athens. In 399 BCE, he was charged with impiety and corrupting the youth and subsequently sentenced to death by drinking poison.

In the end, Socrates' journey serves as a cautionary tale about the limits of individual agency within societal systems resistant to change. Despite his self-awareness, personal values, beliefs, principles, and actions aligned with his dreams and objectives, external forces proved insurmountable, resulting in his untimely demise and the failure to effect the societal transformation he sought.

Socrates' story underscores the complexity and unpredictability of human endeavors, highlighting the importance of considering not only individual agency but also the broader socio-political context in which one operates.

These two stories demonstrate that even if the right building blocks are well understood and used by massively self-aware and reflected individuals, they could lead to both successful and unsuccessful outcomes. This comes from the fact that all these blocks interact continuously in a very dynamic and complex way. This is what we will address in this section, presenting more in detail "The Gray Spot" model and the way to navigate through it while searching for happiness.

7.1 Foundations of Happiness: Understanding and Cultivating Supporting Pillars

---

"The secret of happiness, you see, is not found in seeking more, but in developing the capacity to enjoy less."

Socrates - Ancient Greek philosopher

Objectives of the section

Explore the concept of "happiness supporting pillars," providing insights into the key aspects of life that contribute to happiness and stability. It offers guidance on identifying, nurturing, and maintaining these pillars to achieve a balanced and fulfilling life.

Key topics

UNDERSTAND THE CONCEPT OF HAPPINESS-SUPPORTING PILLARS - This delves into the metaphor of life as a structure supported by pillars, each representing different facets. It emphasizes the importance of maintaining a balance between the quantity and quality of these pillars to ensure stability and happiness.

IDENTIFY AND CULTIVATE KEY PILLARS - Identify the essential pillars that contribute to a stable and fulfilling life, highlighting various contributing aspects and providing guidance on nurturing these pillars to enhance overall well-being.

My life crisis began with the remnants of my "self" buried within the grey spot of my marriage. Barely alive, it fought for liberation, struggling to break free. And eventually, it did. However, my free "self" was small and weak, with almost nothing to lean on. Thus, it quickly searched for a pillar of support and found it - in the form of another man. That was, unfortunately, before confronting my husband about my unhappiness, as my "self" was still far too fragile for any honest dialogue.

Though not a physical love affair, based only on video calls and text messages, the relationship held profound significance. In a way, it was the most beautiful thing that had happened to me in many years. It offered understanding, deep conversations, and respect, accompanied by fluttering butterflies. Yet, I felt great despair and profound unhappiness. I found myself ensnared in a triangle of secrecy and deceit and before long, my husband caught me in my lies about "the other man." I had to decide to stay or leave my marriage, but I was not able to do so. I was trapped in this clandestine triangle for over a year – desperate and unable to decide on which way to take. It was a burden for all of us involved.

In time, I realized why I struggled to decide — my "self" was not stable enough without the supporting pillar of my marriage and was in danger of collapsing without it, yet the pillar alone had become insufficient, so I needed a second pillar which I found in the form of the other relationship. I was on the precipice of another dependency, another gray spot.

Refusing this path, I wanted to address the root cause of the issue. I wanted to find other supporting pillars, not make myself dependent on just one (or two) love relationships. I painted my "house of pillars," recognizing the dearth beyond the two main pillars. However, there were some pre-existing smaller pillars that were not supported yet and that I could maybe build on - my family, my best friend, a new connection with a colleague and sports. I even allowed myself to play religious songs on the piano again and to pray.

I had grown up believing in God and was ashamed of this belief for a long time. It was not accepted in the gray spot of my marriage and vanished within it. Thus, I started going to my family and friends more and more on my own and opening up to them. For years, I had shied away not only from simple basic things, like driving a car by myself (which in itself is isolating) but also from expressing myself outside the confines of my marriage. Gradually, I began to open up to my loved ones, a process that took months. Only then, with a more stable foundation of multiple pillars, could I make a free decision. I made the agonizing decision to leave my marriage—a decision I had once deemed impossible.

Imagine your life as a dynamic edifice, with a foundation supporting a platform representing happiness in life. This foundation relies on pillars, each symbolizing a facet of your life – relationships, career, health, hobbies, and more. The number of pillars reflects your adaptability, while their quality indicates how effectively they maintain the stability of your life.

Now, envision consistently nurturing these pillars, reinforcing them through continual personal growth and adaptation. High-quality pillars resemble well-forged steel beams, robust and resilient, while an ample quantity ensures a sturdy framework (Figure 2).

As life inevitably progresses, the key to sustaining happiness lies in maintaining the stability of your structure, supported by these strategically placed pillars. The balance between quantity and quality ensures that your equilibrium remains resilient, capable of withstanding unforeseen changes and challenges, thus preserving the harmony in your life, by ensuring stability of the happiness dynamic platform.

Figure 2: Visualization of a stable and well-balanced "happiness pillar" structure

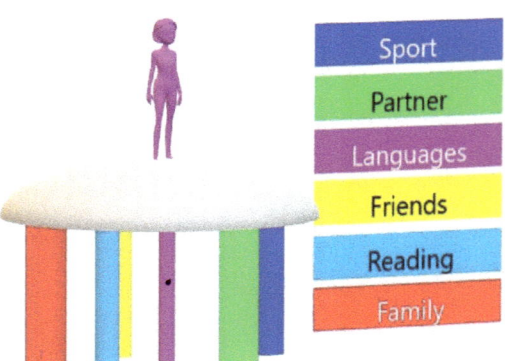

If this balance falters due to weakened or missing pillars – perhaps through a breakup, injury, or neglecting important aspects of life – the stability of your life's structure is jeopardized. Without adequate pillars, the metaphorical happiness ceiling may begin to tilt (Figure 3), eventually collapsing if control is not regained (Figure 4).

Figure 3: Pillar structure facing the challenge of weakened or missing pillars, posing a threat to the stability of one's life happiness

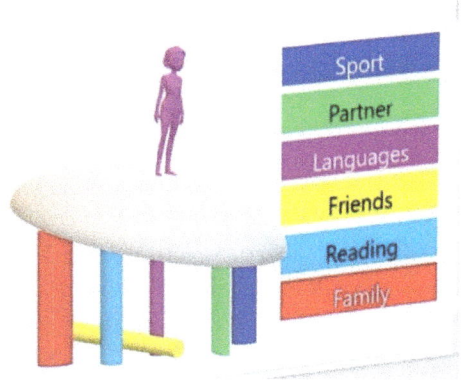

Figure 4: Collapsed pillar structure resulting from a failure to uphold an adequate quantity and strength of the remaining pillars necessary to bear the weight of life

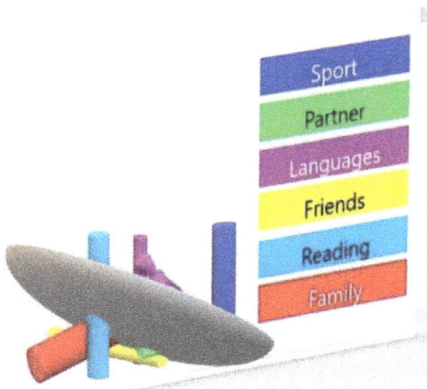

To optimally balance quantity and quality in maintaining stability amid life's uncertainties, it is important to adopt a proactive approach and to regularly reassess and adjust the pillars based on evolving life circumstances. Attention to pillar development, deployment, and reinforcement becomes crucial, mirroring the ongoing effort needed to sustain life's equilibrium and secure the happiness platform in its place.

In essence, to maintain a resilient life ceiling, cultivate a diverse set of pillars by identifying key priorities and interests. Focus on developing a few high-quality pillars that align with core values and provide strong support. Simultaneously, have enough of them to ensure adaptability to unforeseen changes. Strike a balance by having enough pillars for resilience and diversity while ensuring each pillar is well-constructed and robust. This approach enhances your ability to maintain stability amidst life's changes, fostering a dynamic equilibrium and is achieved by nurturing a growth mindset, building a strong support system, and staying committed to personal development. It will enable adjusting your pillars as needed, reinforcing the existing ones with resilience and determination, and adding new ones as needed.

While individual preferences may vary from person to person, defining personal key pillars is best done by listening to core values to set meaningful goals and by regularly reflecting on your life priorities to adjust and realign them with your aspirations.

Below are some essential elements that frequently foster a stable, fulfilling, and vibrant life, emphasizing factors that contribute to overall well-being, fulfillment, and lasting satisfaction. These elements can serve as a foundation for defining your personal pillars. You will observe that many of them are intricately linked to the discussions of Sections 6.3 and 6.4, which centered on values and principles.

Well-being

- Physical Well-being
    - Health and Fitness: Regular exercise, a balanced diet, and sufficient sleep contribute to overall well-being.
- Mental and Emotional Health
    - Mindfulness and Stress Management: Practices such as meditation, mindfulness, and stress reduction techniques can enhance mental well-being.

Financial Stability

- Budgeting and Financial Planning: Responsible financial management, including budgeting and saving, helps maintain stability and security.
- Investing: Smart investments can contribute to long-term financial growth and security.

Meaningful relationships

- Invest time and energy in building, maintaining and nurturing meaningful relationships with family and friends. Strong social connections contribute significantly to happiness and support.
- Community Involvement, engaging and offering time and skills in community activities and contributing to causes beyond oneself fosters a sense of purpose.

Personal Development

- Continuous Learning: Embracing a mindset of continuous learning and personal growth enhances skills, knowledge, and adaptability.

Work-Life Balance

- Career Satisfaction: Pursuing a fulfilling career that aligns with personal values and interests contributes to overall life satisfaction.
- Leisure, hobbies and recreation: Balancing work with hobbies, relaxation, and recreation ensures a well-rounded lifestyle.
- Creativity: Expressing creativity, whether through art, writing, or music, can be a source of joy.

Spirituality and Purpose

- Spiritual Connection - For some, cultivating a sense of spirituality or connection to a higher purpose adds depth and meaning to life.

Maintaining balance involves regular reflection and adjustment to align with personal values and goals. Skills such as simplifying life, living in the present, contributing to others, adaptability and resilience, and gratitude support this process. Diving deeper, the following strategies could prove advantageous in establishing a meaningful and resilient foundation for happiness:

Simplify and Declutter

- Streamline your life by decluttering both physically and mentally. Simplifying your surroundings and commitments can reduce stress and create space for what truly matters.

Live in the Present

- Practice mindfulness and focus on the present moment. Enjoy and fully engage in your experiences without being overly preoccupied with the past or future.

Contribute to Others

- Engage in activities that contribute to the well-being of others. Acts of kindness and meaningful contributions to your community can bring a sense of fulfillment.

Adaptability and Resilience

- Developing the ability to overcome challenges and solve problems enhances resilience.
- Being open to change and adapting to new circumstances promotes long-term stability.

Practice Gratitude

- Cultivate a habit of gratitude. Acknowledge and appreciate the positive aspects of your life regularly.

Remember, what matters varies for each person. Stay intentional in your choices, focusing on aspects contributing most to well-being and fulfilment. Finally, regular self-reflection ensures staying on course as priorities evolve.

My personal pillars

Reflecting on my guiding values delineated in Section 6.3.1, my personal principles outlined in Section 6.4.1, and the resultant goals and actions detailed in Section 6.6.1, the foundation of my personal life currently rests upon the following pillars. Notably, I have intentionally integrated the pursuit of personal development into aspects concerning well-being and work-life balance, as I realized that it aligns with my core values and permeates much of my daily endeavors.

Spirituality and Purpose:

- Contemplating happiness and the significance of existence, and documenting my reflections, including adherence to the principles of "The Gray Spot."

Meaningful Relationships:

- Nurturing familial bonds by fostering close connections with my daughters and former spouse, centered on shared interests.
- Strengthening and cultivating trust and openness with my partner.

Well-being / Personal Development:

- Physical: Engaging in fitness training and adhering to a balanced diet to sustain optimal physical health.
- Mental: Enhancing my breadth of knowledge and embracing new subject matters through reading, exposure to various media, and interaction with mindful individuals.

Work-Life Balance / Personal Development:

- Advancing in my professional journey and fostering career growth in line with my personal values.
- Pursuing diverse hobbies, such as scuba diving and musical endeavors like songwriting and drumming in a rock band, to foster creativity, mindfulness, and personal growth.

7.2 "The Gray Spot": Harmonizing individuality with unity in relationships

Objectives of the section

Explore the delicate balance between maintaining individuality and fostering unity within relationships, acknowledging the benefits and drawbacks of both aspects and providing insights into navigating this balance effectively.

Key topics

MAINTAINING INDIVIDUAL IDENTITIES - Discuss the advantages and disadvantages of preserving individuality within relationships, emphasizing strengthened connections, healthy autonomy, and effective conflict resolution.

OPTIMIZING UNITY - Examine the benefits of merging identities within relationships while maintaining balance, including enhanced unity, greater harmony, and simplified communication.

As we delved into Section 7.1, constructing the foundational pillars of our happiness, we have come to a profound realization: the pursuit of happiness hinges on effectively navigating two fundamental realms simultaneously.

Firstly, there is the intricate landscape of the personal self. As spotlighted in Section 6.1 with the "Selfishness" model, at our core, our individuality defines us, encapsulating our strengths, weaknesses, values, beliefs, and unique communication styles. It is through this lens that we understand our past, present, and aspirations for the future.

Secondly, we are inherently social beings, drawn to and by others. Our survival and growth intertwine with the web of connections we weave, be it with family, friends, partners, or colleagues. These relationships thrive on trust, honesty, communication, shared objectives, mutual respect, empathy, and understanding.

Fostering these positive dynamics demands transparent sharing of emotions, needs, experiences and expectations, time investment in relationships, clear boundaries, collaboration, constructive conflict resolution, and unwavering mutual support. While each relationship possesses its nuances, these principles form the bedrock of any meaningful connection.

Eddie Cantor, American comedian, singer, actor, and songwriter, once quipped, "Marriage is an attempt to solve problems together which you didn't even have when you were on your own." Indeed, our social nature propels us towards companionship, driven by various factors ranging from physical attraction to shared values. While initial attraction may be rooted in singular factors, including physical appearance, personality traits, shared interests or values, emotional connection, intellectual stimulation, and compatibility in goals or lifestyles, relationships evolve into complex, nonlinear journeys, shaping and reshaping involved individuals and the bond they share. But before delving into this evolution, it is crucial to examine the repercussions—both positive and negative—of maintaining or sacrificing individual identities within a relationship.

These two aspects are essentially two sides of the same coin, each presenting advantages and drawbacks that must be managed simultaneously to achieve optimal balance for both individuals and the relationship. Maintaining individual identities within a relationship offers several benefits:

- *Strengthened connection*: Embracing individual identities enriches the relationship by incorporating diverse perspectives, interests, and strengths. Each person's uniqueness adds depth to the bond, fostering understanding and appreciation.
- *Healthy autonomy*: Both partners maintain the freedom to pursue personal growth, hobbies, and friendships outside the relationship. This autonomy fosters independence and fulfilment, contributing to overall well-being.
- *Conflict resolution*: While preserving separate identities may introduce differences in values or lifestyles, it also presents opportunities for growth. Effective communication and compromise are essential for navigating these disparities, ultimately strengthening the relationship.

However, pushing individuality too far can also lead to significant drawbacks:

- *Impaired connection*: Rigidly maintaining individual identities may hinder the development of a deep connection between partners. Prioritizing personal interests and perspectives could impede understanding and empathy, leading to emotional distance and discord.
- *Autonomy challenges*: While upholding separate identities promotes autonomy, it may also spark tension and conflicts within the relationship. Divergent goals and priorities could result in power struggles and feelings of neglect or resentment.
- *Difficulty in conflict resolution*: Conflicts stemming from differing values or lifestyles can pose challenges when partners strongly identify with their individuality. Effective communication and compromise become more challenging as each person prioritizes their own needs and preferences, potentially prolonging conflicts.

Conversely, sacrificing one's individual identity in favor of the relationship comes with its own set of drawbacks:

- *Co-dependency*: When individual identities diminish within the relationship, a harmful dependency can emerge. Each partner's self-worth becomes excessively reliant on the other, fostering insecurity and emotional instability.
- *Loss of fulfilment*: Neglecting personal interests and goals may lead to stagnation or emptiness. This lack of fulfilment can breed resentment or dissatisfaction within the relationship, undermining its stability.
- *Conflict avoidance*: Merged identities might tempt partners to suppress individual needs to maintain harmony, potentially masking underlying issues and fostering resentment.

Nevertheless, managing this aspect properly and together can yield significant benefits for the relationship:

- *Enhanced unity*: Surrendering individual identities can foster a deeper sense of unity within the relationship. Prioritizing collective goals and interests over personal ones may lead to a stronger bond built on shared experiences and mutual support.
- *Greater harmony*: Without the excessive burden of personal ambitions and desires, couples may find it easier to navigate conflicts and disagreements. Aligning their identities more closely can foster a harmonious atmosphere where compromise prevails.
- *Simplified communication*: Merged identities streamline communication, eliminating the need to negotiate individual preferences and priorities. This simplification can result in clearer, more efficient interactions and decision-making processes.

The path to a harmonious balance between individuality and unity necessitates integrating key aspects, fostering open communication, understanding, and continually adjusting as identities evolve. Ultimately, it is through this delicate equilibrium that enduring and fulfilling relationships are forged.

We will now outline a conceivable process delineating the various stages involved in forming, developing, and evolving interpersonal connections. All the ideas elaborated upon in Section 6, as well as the "happiness supporting pillars" model presented in Section 7.1, will serve as foundational elements to be integrated into this model. Subsequently, the following section 7.3 will concentrate on delineating steps to navigate the model effectively and derive maximum benefit from it.

Figure 5 represents a visualization of the progression of positive energy and emotions as they advance through the various phases of the model. This acts as a catalyst for personal happiness and fulfilment.

Figure 5 : Visualization of the evolution of the positive energy and emotions level in its different phases

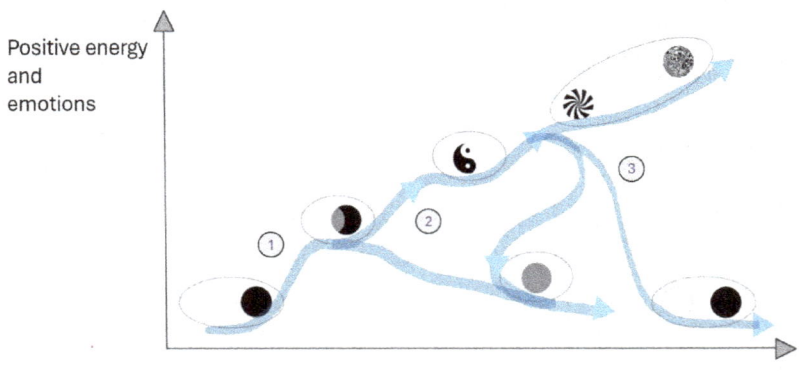

The three main phases that we identified are described in detail here, starting from the individual him/herself.

Initial state *– The individual – "1"*

The individual stands alone, characterized by his/her distinct traits and qualities as we have navigated through in Section 6.

Phase 1 *– First contact – From "1" + "1" to "1+1=2"*

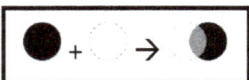

141

Individuals intersect with others, drawn together by specific elements such as:

- Common interests
- Similar viewpoints and/or perspectives
- Physical attraction

Initially, their individual identities remain intact, with only certain interests shared, before further development ensues.

This is, for instance, the case for romantic partnerships characterized by Initial attraction and a limited commitment.

Phase 2 – *Connecting and Progressing* – From "1+1=2" to "1+1=3" or "1+1=1"

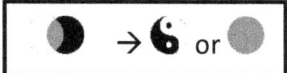

As shared interests deepen, relationships evolve. This progression may lead to different scenarios:

- The emergence of synergistic behaviors while preserving individual identities. A new relational identity emerges alongside personal identities, blending their specificities without eroding individualities. This marks a transition to a new phase, blending identities – "1+1=3" – which could be visualized as a "Yin yang" structure. However, while still in its infancy, this phase requires careful integration to avoid regression to the initial connection state – "1+1=2" – or "The Gray Spot" state – "1+1=1" (as detailed below).

  or:

- The formation of a new relational identity that absorbs or assimilates the individual identities, resulting in a fusion where distinctions blur – "1+1=1" – "The Gray Spot" state. This is, in particular, characterized by the following:

- Systematic joint activities
- Intense emotional investment
- Compromises to avoid conflict
- A desire for sameness and unity
- Resistance to judgment and disagreement
- Sacrifices of personal expectations

While initially perceived as ideal, such relationships risk co-dependency and the loss of individuality, hindering happiness in the long term.

Phase 3 – *Optimizing and subliming* – From "1+1=3" to "1+1= ∞" or "1+1=1" or "1" + "1"

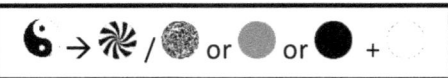

As relationships progress, expectations rise, demanding more nuanced interactions and communication to address conflicts constructively. Here again, there are multiple possible scenarios which require attention:

- "1+1= ∞": Achieving a delicate balance between the relationship and individual identities, nurturing both. This state is neither uniquely defined nor fixed in time; it will likely continue evolving, maintaining and refining the intricacies of the selves within the relationship. It involves a complex set of interactions:
  - Sharing important experiences while preserving personal space
  - Maintaining diverse perspectives harmoniously
  - Emotionally investing in the relationship without sacrificing autonomy
  - Making conscious compromises without significant negative impacts
  - Prioritizing mutual understanding and happiness
  - Setting clear and aligned expectations

- Managing conflicts constructively
- Maintaining loose boundaries
- Respecting differences without imposing conformity
- Adopting a flexible, positive attitude

or:

- "1+1=1": As interactions intensify, the boundary between individual identities and the relationship blurs, potentially leading to "The Gray Spot" situation characterized by, as described here above:
  - Strong emotional fusion
  - Excessive compromises
  - The desire for complete unity
  - Avoidance of conflicts

or:

- "1" + "1": The relationship identity dissipates under the pressure of increasing complexity, leaving only the initial individual identities. Once perceived synergies diminish, the individuals' identities diverge until getting back to the initial state of two separate individuals.

Although "1+1= ∞" might be perceived as the ultimate desired outcome, it is essential to acknowledge the accompanying risks, particularly the possibility of individual identities being absorbed into the relationship, especially as emotions and feelings intensify and the relationship becomes more intricate. It is imperative to remain vigilant to prevent this scenario and uphold equilibrium.

Key factors to consider and address consistently include:

- Recognizing vulnerable areas and sources of instability
- Evaluating the preservation of individuality
- Monitoring the relationship's stability
- Maintaining balanced dynamics

Optimal navigation along this evolutionary path towards happiness entails understanding and managing complex, interconnected factors, including those addressed within "The Gray Spot":

- Clarifying personal values and aspirations
- Cultivating emotional intelligence
- Nurturing healthy relationships, considering various dynamics (romantic, familial, social, professional)
- Emphasizing elements such as unconditional love, trust, and interdependency
- Exploring existential questions and belonging

While this book touches upon some of the fundamental aspects, future iterations of "The Gray Spot" will delve deeper into specific dynamics and strategies.

7.3 Implementing "The Gray Spot" strategies: A roadmap to personal evolution

Objectives of the section

Outline the process of navigating "The Gray Spot," which involves understanding its complexity and implementing strategies for personal evolution and happiness.

Key topics

UNDERSTANDING COMPLEXITY - Discuss how "The Gray Spot" represents a complex process involving various interconnected components.

PRACTICAL APPLICATION - Provide practical steps for synthesizing knowledge about oneself, establishing personal pillars, and initiating the journey of self-discovery and evolution.

RISK MITIGATION – Identify common risks and pitfalls related to self-awareness, emotional intelligence, goal setting, relationships, and adaptation, offering mitigation strategies to address them effectively.

Maya had always felt like she was wandering through life, navigating a sea of uncertainty and discontent. Despite her best efforts, she could not seem to find her footing or grasp a sense of lasting happiness. But then she stumbled upon a roadmap to personal evolution, "The Gray Spot" strategies, which promised to illuminate her path toward fulfilment.

Understanding Complexity

Maya realized that happiness was not a simple destination; it was a multifaceted journey intertwined with various interconnected components. Just like the emergent properties in biological, social, economic, and environmental systems, her happiness stemmed from the intricate relationships among her past, present, and future selves.

Practical Application

Armed with this understanding, Maya delved into the practical steps outlined in the roadmap. She reflected on her past, identifying pivotal events, relationships, and emotions that shaped her. Determining her personal values and formulating a code of principles provided her with a compass to navigate life's complexities. With clarity on her objectives and aspirations, Maya established practical goals and corresponding actions to propel her forward.

Make it Happen

Constructing her personal pillar structure served as a foundation for Maya's journey. She conducted regular sanity checks, ensuring alignment with her values, principles, and goals. Maya understood the importance of surrounding herself with supportive individuals and environments conducive to her growth.

Transitioning from an individual to a part of a larger system, Maya embraced the dynamics of positive energy and momentum. She identified key drivers for enhancement and stability while remaining transparent with her emotions and those of others. Maya committed to continuous improvement, recognizing that every action, no matter how small, contributed to her evolution.

Navigating Peaks and Valleys

Maya's journey was not without its challenges. There were moments of self-doubt, setbacks, and unforeseen obstacles. However, she learned to pivot and bifurcate, optimizing her personal evolution in the face of adversity. By strategizing optimal transitions and managing the speed of change, Maya ensured that her journey remained fluid yet grounded.

Iterative Evolution

Maya embraced the iterative nature of her journey, understanding that personal evolution had no clear finish line. She updated her "Gray Spot" model regularly, recalibrating her actions and priorities based on daily reflections. Each constraint, roadblock, or hiccup became an opportunity for learning and growth, reinforcing her resilience along the way.

Mitigating Risks and Pitfalls

Throughout her journey, Maya remained vigilant against common risks and pitfalls. She cultivated self-awareness, emotional intelligence, and goal-setting to mitigate potential conflicts and stress. Maya prioritized open communication, boundary-setting, and supportive connections, guarding against toxic relationships that could impede her progress.

Embracing Change and Adaptability

Maya faced her fears of change head-on, embracing growth as an opportunity for self-discovery. She adopted a holistic approach, recognizing the interconnectedness of life's aspects and prioritizing adaptability in her personal model. By cultivating a growth mindset and remaining open to new experiences, Maya navigated life's challenges with confidence and purpose.

As Maya danced to her own rhythm, she realized that happiness was not a destination to reach but a way of life to embrace. With each step forward, she celebrated her evolution, knowing that the floor was hers to enjoy.

We have traversed the various components comprising "The Gray Spot," delving into the individual, the relationships, and their contributions to personal happiness. Now, the focus shifts to bringing this understanding to life, extracting the utmost from our pursuit of happiness. A pivotal aspect involves acknowledging the complexity of this process, which diverges from mere summation in several critical ways. While individual elements may appear straightforward in isolation, when intertwined into a complex process, emergent properties arise that elude prediction based solely on the examination of individual components. Analogous complex phenomena permeate our surroundings and societies:

- *Biological systems*, where an organism's behavior surpasses the sum of its constituent cells, leading for example, in the case of the brain, to the emergent property of consciousness from neural connections.
- *Social systems*, where cultural norms, political movements, and economic trends emerge from interactions among individuals within related societies or institutions, are shaped by historical, cultural, and environmental factors.
- *Economic systems*, where inflation, unemployment rates, and market crashes stem from interactions and feedback loops involving various components such as individuals, businesses, governments, and financial markets.
- *Environmental ecosystems*, where the dynamics depend on intricate relationships among plant species, soil microorganisms, and climatic conditions, are influenced by nutrient cycling, energy flow, and biodiversity.

As elucidated in this book, the complexity of "The Gray Spot" arises from the intimate interplay of the components discussed in Section 6, serving as both the starting point and a prerequisite for personal evolution. These components contribute to a deeper understanding of oneself and the desired self.

Understanding one's past, present, and future

1. Understand where you come from - Learn from your past from events, environments, relationships, and related emotions.

2. Determining personal values.
3. Formulating a personal code or principles.
4. Clarifying life objectives, dreams, and aspirations.
5. Establishing practical objectives and corresponding actions.

The subsequent phase entails synthesizing this knowledge and ensuring its practical application in daily life.

Make it happen

1. Constructing a personal pillar structure (Section 7.1).
2. Conducting a sanity check to evaluate the completeness and adjustability of the structure in alignment with values, principles, and goals. Namely:
   a. What do I need to reach my goals?
   b. What can I get from myself independently of others?
   c. What can I get from the people around me? Family, friends, social groups or colleagues
   d. What do I additionally need?
   e. Who could provide me with this?

Before embarking on navigation through the sea of "The Gray Spot," comprehending the essence of the model, owning it, and tailoring it to individual needs and specificities are imperative.

Understand, clarify and own your personal (adapted if needed) version of the "Gray Spot" model.

Subsequently, one is primed to:

Start your self-discovery and evolution journey

1. Act consistently on defined actions to fortify pillars and progress toward fulfilment.
2. Identify and engage with supportive individuals, activities, and environments conducive to goal achievement.

As the journey unfolds, transitioning from an individual to a constituent of a larger system with intricate interfaces and relationships becomes apparent.

Transition from solitary wanderer to an integral part of an organism

1. Initiate dynamics by leveraging positive initial energy and momentum.
2. Enhance and stabilize through key drivers.
3. Identify factors indicative of structural damage, including risks from relationships, loss of focus, or resurgence of negative aspects from the past. This can be triggered on a daily basis by asking the following questions to yourself:
    a. How am I doing with myself (stabilize the self)?
    b. How am I doing with you (stabilize the partnerships)?
    c. How am I doing with others (stabilize the relationships)?

   and to others:

    d. How are you doing with yourself (stabilize others' self)?
    e. How are you doing with me (stabilize the partnerships)?
    f. How are you doing with others (stabilize the relationships)?
4. Be transparent with your feelings and emotions as well as the ones from others. This is pivotal to address the key hurdles towards happiness.
5. Act to continuously improve and maintain stability – everyday, everything – nothing is trivial and should be negligible.
6. Manage failure reactively and together – learn continuously.

During your journey, you will not only face extraordinary discoveries about yourself, others and the world surrounding you, but also some constraints, roadblocks and hiccups which will put a lot in question. This is part of the discovery and development cycle and should not be taken as reasons to give up but more as opportunities to learn and to adjust your actions, priorities and focus areas as needed. In such situations, it is critical to be able to:

Pivot and bifurcate to optimize your personal evolution and your life journey.

1. Identify the key drivers that will enable adjusting and/or pivoting your actions and priorities.
2. Strategize optimal transitions from the current to the future state, including what will be the pros and cons, what will be won and lost, and what will be the consequences on your life pillars so that stability is ensured and reinforced.
3. Manage the speed of change to guarantee that the adjustments occur fast enough but do not jeopardize the rest of the pillars, and make sure that potential short-term wins do not screen out the long-term objectives.

Even if starting the journey is critical, it is even more important to understand that the process is an iterative one and that there is no clear finish line but only a continuous evolution, development, and search for happiness. Based on the risks and opportunities identified on a daily basis, you need to:

Update your personal "Gray Spot" model

1. Go recursively through the process described here above, focusing on the points that resonate and make the most sense to you.

This methodology will foster your resilience, fortifying you to navigate life's peaks and valleys with strength, seizing every opportunity for personal and collective growth. Throughout this journey, you will cultivate robust self-confidence, enabling you to actively manage forthcoming challenges and maintain mastery over your "Gray Spot" model. However, it is crucial to remain vigilant, acknowledging the perpetual risks of reverting to old habits or facing unforeseen events that could exert significant, uncontrollable impacts on both you and your surroundings.

Recognizing and mitigating risks and pitfalls

Below are some risks that are likely to impact your progression within "The Gray Spot" model, along with proposed strategies to mitigate or minimize their potential negative effects.

Linked with personal self - Enhancing self-awareness, emotional intelligence, and goal-setting

Risk 1: Inadequate self-awareness may lead to decisions conflicting with personal values, interests, or strengths.

Mitigation: Engage in self-reflection through journaling, meditation, or therapy. Seek feedback from trusted sources and invest time in activities to understand passions and weaknesses.

Risk 2: Ignoring Emotions - Neglecting emotions can cause stress and disconnection from oneself.

Mitigation: Practice mindfulness to acknowledge emotions without judgment. Develop emotional intelligence by recognizing and expressing feelings constructively and in healthy ways, such as through art, exercise, or talking with supportive individuals.

Risk 3: Unrealistic Goals - Setting overly ambitious goals can result in frustration and burnout.

Mitigation: Establish SMART (Specific, Measurable, Achievable, Relevant, Time-bound) goals, break them into achievable steps, and celebrate milestones for sustained motivation. Regularly review and adjust your goals based on progress and feedback-

Risk 4: Settling for Low Goals - Easy goals may lead to stagnation and hinder personal growth.

Mitigation: Pursue challenging goals, embrace continuous learning, and surround oneself with supportive individuals who are inspiring and encourage excellence.

Linked with relationships - Fostering open communication, boundary-setting, and supportive connections

Risk 5: Disregarding others' perspectives - Ignoring feedback hampers growth and collaboration.

Mitigation: Practice active listening, seek diverse viewpoints, be open to constructive criticism and feedback, and build supportive relationships based on mutual respect and trust.

Risk 6: Toxic relationships - Surrounding oneself with negativity impedes progress and happiness.

Mitigation: Evaluate relationships regularly, set boundaries with individuals who drain your energy or undermine your goals, and nurture connections with like-minded individuals.

Linked with "The Gray Spot" model - Embracing change, holistic development, and adaptability.

Risk 7: Fear of change - Resistance to change stifles personal development and might prevent reaching the next stage of happiness.

Mitigation: Embrace change as an opportunity for growth, practice resilience, and seek support from trusted friends, family, or professionals during transitions and times of uncertainty

Risk 8: Overlooking Interconnections - Neglecting the interconnectedness of life aspects might lead to imbalance.

Mitigation: Adopt a holistic approach considering how different areas of your life (e.g., health, relationships, career) influence one another, prioritize values, and integrate different dimensions for sustainable growth rather than pursuing growth in isolation.

Risk 9: Failure to Adapt - Stagnation occurs without adapting personal models (like your personal "Gray Spot" model)

Mitigation: Embrace a growth mindset, regularly reassess beliefs, values and goals and remain open to new experiences and perspectives for continual improvement. Cultivate flexibility and adaptability in your approach to navigating life's challenges and opportunities.

Equipped with this knowledge, you are then encouraged to integrate these principles into your daily life, seizing the opportunity to dance to your own rhythm with confidence and purpose. Enjoy it! The floor is yours!

8 Epilogue – Beyond "The Gray Spot" – Jump in!

Having made the toughest decision of my life—parting ways with my husband—I moved out. I adopted two baby cats and started to build my own life. Those around me told me that I was thriving. I found it hard to see, as I cried daily for months. I missed my husband and the familiarity of the gray spot. Yet, I knew returning was no longer possible. As a liberated adult woman, I simply no longer fit into that small gray spot.

Now I can say that I am happy. Not always, but overall. I have cultivated some wonderful relationships with people who are important to me, including a friendship with my soon-to-be ex-husband. My pursuits in sports, music, faith, and the companionship of my cats make me feel stable and happy. The love affair from the separation period has gradually evolved into a profound romantic relationship characterized by love, respect, freedom and individuality. We do not live together yet and I think I need it that way for a while to avoid getting back into another gray spot.

And one thing makes me especially happy: I know what I like again. This may seem trivial for some, but for me, it is a treasure. For my last birthday, my father asked me what I wanted as a present. Without much hesitation, I knew—a vibrant, oversized birthday cake for my celebration. Though seemingly irrational, it was what I really wanted and not what I thought others would expect me to want. Cutting this cake together with my new partner, surrounded by my family and friends, was a beautiful and happy moment symbolic of having found my own colorful identity again.

While in the initial months of my self-discovery journey, I experienced a continuous descent into what felt like hell. The lack of answers to my myriad questions pushed me further into what seemed like an inescapable dead end. As I delved deeper into self-introspection, I grappled with extremely dark thoughts about life's meaning and whether happiness was even attainable. Questions like "Why am I here?" and "Am I worth anything?" plagued my mind.

Refusing to evade life without finding answers, I focused on clarifying the questions I needed to ask myself. I embarked on a journey to rediscover myself beyond the protective shell I had meticulously crafted over the years. I spent countless evenings and weekends contemplating, reading books, and penning my darkest thoughts into song lyrics. I also strengthened interactions with individuals whom I could support, leveraging my growing understanding of human psychology and societal complexities.

Gradually, patterns began to emerge, connecting my past experiences to my present self. From them, I gained invaluable insights into what my values were and started to put words on some of the strong emotions I had been keeping locked inside me for years. Taking the example of my separation and its impact on my family, I was able to connect with the one who would become my partner in life and to consolidate all these pieces until "The Gray Spot" model emerged, first adapted for couples and then more generally linked with any type of relationship and life evolution of individuals.

Furthermore, my commitment to self-improvement led me to realize that I had kept on reinforcing my life-supporting pillars without even noticing it. It started with reading and writing to support my reflections, carrying out my scuba diver advanced certification, and keeping on investing myself within our rock band as the main songwriter and drummer, which helped me maintain contacts with my ex-wife (who is the singer in the band) and served as a base for later reinforcing the dynamics of our new familial structure. All this enabled me to progress in the direction of accepting who I really was and generate increased resilience while starting to focus on what really mattered to me, independently of what society was indirectly expecting from me.

This relief from the pressure from the external world and the new refocus on my key priorities allowed me to start progressing in the direction of discovering what happiness could mean. This translated into newfound confidence to do what was good for me and a reduction of the fear of others' opinions. As a consequence, I could continue opening up to myself as well as to others, further reinforcing the aspects of the familial bonds that were important to me and increasing my professional networking with like-minded and challenging people. The connection I developed with my emotions and feelings allowed me to reduce my need to control my reactions which had been putting pressure on me and others in the past, but to act mainly on what was important to me and the ones dear to me.

This new me, even if he still requires pursuing the direction of better knowing and reinforcing himself, enabled me to recently cope with unexpected changes much more easily, accept others for who they are and focus on what they can bring me as well as what I can bring them. These first important changes reflected in some positive outcomes which contributed to making me realize what happiness could look like. Namely:

- Accompanying my daughters with the course of their first steps in their adult lives, in close collaboration with my ex-wife with whom we have reinforced our relationship in the new environment.
- Building a strong relationship with my new partner, ensuring that we respect our differences in addition to consolidating a common identity.
- Being able to manage positively the recent loss of my job after realizing that my principles and values were not aligned with the ones demonstrated by the organization I was working for.

Looking back, these are things I would have been unable to accomplish some years ago. It encourages me to continue what I have initiated, with the ambition to be able to say on my deathbed that I reached a sense of happiness. The emotions I experience when thinking strongly about the examples above, or which sometimes overwhelm me, continuously remind me that even if I am on the right track, I should remain conscious that "The Gray Spot" is never far away, waiting in the shadows to dissolve my personal identity into some illusory ideal relationship, and nothing should be considered as given. I then take some time to reflect on the good progress I have made and step back into my journey towards happiness.

When discussions began, my aim was to delve into self-understanding and explore avenues for managing one's life to mitigate unhappiness and, ideally, cultivate a sense of contentment. As conversations and interactions on the topic progressed, I found that synthesizing my thoughts and maintaining alignment propelled me beyond mere post-mortems of potential buried love relationships. Gradually, this endeavor morphed into a broader mission: unravelling the core elements of human happiness. I then dedicated myself to consolidating my evolving ideas and insights on the subject, leading to a higher collective purpose, vision, and mission which crystallized as follows and will serve as the foundation for my forthcoming focus and the further development of the "Gray Spot" concept and approach:

Purpose: To empower individuals on a transformative journey of self-discovery and personal development, facilitating their escape from their "Gray Spot" and celebration of their uniqueness.

Vision: A world where individuals embrace their authentic selves, paint their lives with vibrant colors, and liberate themselves from the confines of "The Gray Spot."

Mission: To furnish practical tools, insights, and guidance for individuals to unearth their authentic selves, reclaim their identity, and lead enriching lives.

This initial endeavor culminated in the creation of the content within this book unified under the banner of "*Escaping The Gray Spot - A Colorful Journey of Self-discovery.*" I view this as a personal odyssey that each individual seeking greater happiness should embark upon independently. I have provided some basic resources within this document to aid you in commencing your own journey.

As you engage with this material, you will discover that your narrative, experiences, and approaches may diverge from what I have described here. I encourage you to leverage as much as resonates with you and remain open to refining and expanding my perspectives, models, and methodologies based on diverse inputs and feedback. I envision a future where this initiative sparks similar introspection in many others, evolving into a community where individuals share their personal victories, challenges, setbacks, and insights, as I firmly believe that the pursuit of happiness is a universal human endeavor that can enrich everyone's lives.

9 References

CHAPTER 4 - Introduction

- "The Essential Drucker: The Best of Sixty Years of Peter Drucker's Essential Writings on Management," Peter F. Drucker, Harper Business, 2001 - A comprehensive collection of Peter Drucker's seminal writings on management, providing insights into effective organizational strategies.
- "The Interpretation of Dreams," Sigmund Freud, Basic Books, 2010 (Originally published in 1899) - Freud's groundbreaking work delving into the analysis of dreams and their significance in understanding the human psyche.

CHAPTER 5 - Happiness – General concepts

Section 5.1 - Looking for happiness

- "A Theory of Human Motivation," Abraham H. Maslow, Sublime Books, 1943 - Maslow's hierarchy of needs theory, proposing a framework for understanding human motivation and fulfilment.
- "Stumbling on Happiness," Daniel Gilbert, Vintage Books, 2007 - Gilbert explores the psychology of happiness, challenging conventional notions and offering insights into the complexities of human contentment.
- "World Happiness Report," John F. Helliwell., Richard Layard., Jeffrey D. Sachs., Jan-Emmanuel De Neve., Lara B. Aknin., & Shun Wang (Eds.), University of Oxford: Wellbeing Research Centre, 2024 - The report explores global happiness trends, factors influencing well-being, and policy implications to enhance citizens' happiness worldwide.
- "The Art of Happiness," Dalai Lama and Howard Cutler, Riverhead Books, 1998 - A collaboration between the Dalai Lama and psychiatrist Howard Cutler, discussing the pursuit of happiness through Buddhist principles and Western psychology.
- "Happiness: A Guide to Developing Life's Most Important Skill," Matthieu Ricard, Little, Brown and Company, 2007 - Ricard, a Buddhist monk, shares perspectives on cultivating happiness and well-being through mindfulness and altruism.
- "The Happiness Hypothesis: Finding Modern Truth in Ancient Wisdom," Jonathan Haidt, Basic Books, 2006 - Haidt examines the intersection of ancient philosophy and modern psychology to uncover insights into human happiness and fulfilment.
- "Bhutan's Gross National Happiness Index: Methods and Data," Centre for Bhutan Studies & GNH Research, Centre for Bhutan Studies, 2012 - A study detailing Bhutan's unique approach to measuring societal well-being through the Gross National Happiness Index.

Section 5.2 - Embarking on the Journey to Inner Harmony: Understanding the Mechanisms of Happiness

- "The Brain: The Story of You," David Eagleman, Vintage Books, 2016 - Eagleman explores the complexities of the human brain, offering insights into how neurological processes shape perceptions and emotions.
- "The Emotional Life of Your Brain: How Its Unique Patterns Affect the Way You Think, Feel, and Live—and How You Can Change Them," Richard J. Davidson and Sharon Begley, Hudson Street Press, 2012 - Davidson and Begley delve into the neuroscience of emotions, highlighting the brain's role in shaping emotional responses and well-being.
- "How Emotions Are Made: The Secret Life of the Brain," Lisa Feldman Barrett, Houghton Mifflin Harcourt, 2017 - Barrett challenges traditional views on emotions, presenting a novel theory on how the brain constructs emotional experiences.
- "Emotional Intelligence: Why It Can Matter More Than IQ," Daniel Goleman, Bantam Books, 1995 - Goleman explores the concept of emotional intelligence and its impact on personal and professional success.

CHAPTER 6 - Who am I and who do I want to be?

Section 6.1 - The Journey of Self-Integration: Navigating the Depths of Human Nature - The "selfishness" model

- "Toward a Psychology of Being," Abraham H. Maslow, Wiley, 1962 - Maslow expands on his hierarchy of needs theory, exploring the concept of self-actualization and the pursuit of personal growth and fulfilment.
- "The Johari Window: A Graphic Model for Interpersonal Relations," Joseph Luft and Harry Ingham, the University of California Western Training Lab, 1955 - The Johari Window model provides a framework for understanding self-awareness and interpersonal communication.
- "The Selfish Gene" by Richard Dawkins, Oxford University Press, 1976 - Dawkins introduces the concept of the selfish gene, exploring how genes drive evolutionary behavior and shape individual survival strategies.
- "The Compassionate Instinct: The Science of Human Goodness" by Dacher Keltner, W. W. Norton & Company, 2010 - Keltner discusses the evolutionary roots of compassion and altruism, challenging the notion of humans as inherently selfish beings.

Section 6.2 - Understanding Your Roots

- "The Child In You: The Breakthrough Method for Bringing Out Your Authentic Self," Stefanie Stahl, J. P. Tarcher, 2006 - Stahl offers insights into understanding and reconnecting with one's authentic self, exploring the impact of childhood experiences on personality development.
- "Living with Intensity: Understanding the Sensitivity, Excitability, and Emotional Development of Gifted Children, Adolescents, and Adults," Susan Daniels and Michael M. Piechowski, Great Potential Press, 2008 - This book provides a comprehensive examination of intensity in gifted individuals across different age groups. It explores the nature of intensity and its impact on various aspects of life and offers practical strategies for parents, educators, and mental health

professionals to support and nurture gifted individuals effectively.

- "Man's Search for Meaning," Viktor E. Frankl, Beacon Press, 1959 - Frankl reflects on his experiences as a Holocaust survivor, proposing that the search for meaning is the primary motivation in human life.
- "12 Rules for Life: An Antidote to Chaos," Jordan Peterson, Penguin Random House Canada, 2018 - Peterson presents twelve principles for living a meaningful and fulfilling life, drawing on psychology, philosophy, and mythology.

Section 6.3 - Unveiling Personal Values

- "Gandhi: An Autobiography – The Story of My Experiments with Truth," Mahatma Gandhi, Beacon Press, 1927 - Gandhi shares his life experiences and philosophy, emphasizing the importance of truth, nonviolence, and compassion.
- "I Am Malala: The Story of the Girl Who Stood Up for Education and Was Shot by the Taliban," Malala Yousafzai and Christina Lamb, Little, Brown and Company, 2013 - Malala recounts her journey as an advocate for girls' education and human rights, embodying values of courage, resilience, and activism.

Section 6.4 - Creating Your Guiding Principles

- "Principles," Ray Dalio, Simon & Schuster, 2017 - Dalio shares his principles for success in life and business based on his experiences as an investor and entrepreneur.
- "Be More Pirate," Sam Conniff Allende, Simon & Schuster UK, 2018 - Allende explores the principles of piracy as a metaphor for disrupting the status quo and fostering social change.
- "Start with Why," Simon Sinek, Portfolio, 2009 - Sinek discusses the importance of starting with a clear sense of purpose, inspiring action and loyalty through understanding the 'why' behind actions.
- "The 5 Dysfunctions of a Team," Patrick Lencioni, Jossey-Bass, 2002 - Lencioni identifies common pitfalls in team dynamics and offers strategies for building cohesive and high-performing teams.

Section 6.5 - Dream Exploration: Unveiling Your Deepest Desires

- "Parting the Waters: America in the King Years 1954-63," Taylor Branch, Simon & Schuster, 1988 - Branch chronicles the Civil Rights Movement in the United States, exploring themes of justice, equality, and social change.
- "Insane Success for Lazy People," Andrii Sedniev, CreateSpace Independent Publishing Platform, 2015 - Sedniev presents strategies for achieving success with minimal effort, challenging conventional notions of productivity and achievement.
- "168 Hours: You Have More Time Than You Think: create a personal list of 100 dreams," Laura Vanderkam, Portfolio, 2010 - Vanderkam offers a practical approach to time management, encouraging readers to prioritize their goals and aspirations.
- "Creative Visualization: Use the Power of Your Imagination to Create What You Want in Your Life," Shakti Gawain, New World Library, 2002 - Gawain explores the practice of creative visualization as a tool for manifesting desires and achieving personal growth.
- "Mindfulness in Plain English," Bhante Henepola Gunaratana, Wisdom Publications, 1991 - Gunaratana provides a straightforward guide to mindfulness meditation, offering techniques for cultivating present-moment awareness and inner peace.

Section 6.6 - Set practical objectives and related actions

- "The 7 Habits of Highly Effective People," Stephen Covey, Free Press, 1989 - Covey presents a holistic approach to personal and professional effectiveness, emphasizing principles of proactive behavior and goal setting.
- "Atomic Habits," James Clear, Avery, 2018 - Clear explores the science of habit formation, offering practical strategies for building and sustaining positive habits.
- "Getting Things Done: The Art of Stress-Free Productivity," David Allen, Penguin Books, 2001 - Allen introduces the GTD (Getting Things Done) method, providing a framework for organizing tasks and achieving stress-free productivity.

CHAPTER 7 – "The Gray Spot" model

- "Long Walk to Freedom," Nelson Mandela, Back Bay Books, 1994 - Mandela recounts his journey as a leader in the struggle against apartheid, embodying principles of resilience, forgiveness, and reconciliation.
- "The Trial and Death of Socrates," Plato (399 BC), John M. Cooper, Translated by G.M.A. Grube, Hackett Publishing Company, 2000 - Plato's dialogue explores the trial and execution of Socrates, raising questions about ethics, justice, and the nature of truth.

Section 7.1 - Foundations of Happiness: Understanding and Cultivating Supporting Pillars

- "Flow: The Psychology of Optimal Experience," Mihaly Csikszentmihalyi, Harper Perennial, 1990 - Csikszentmihalyi introduces the concept of flow, a state of deep engagement and satisfaction that arises from immersive experiences.
- "Mindset: The New Psychology of Success," Carol S. Dweck, Random House, 2006 - Dweck discusses the power of mindset in shaping attitudes toward learning, growth, and achievement.

Section 7.2 - "The Gray Spot": Harmonizing individuality with unity in relationships

- "Designing Your Life: How to Build a Well-Lived, Joyful Life," Bill Burnett and Dave Evans, Knopf, 2016 - Burnett and Evans offer a design thinking approach to life planning, encouraging readers to create meaningful and fulfilling lifestyles.

Section 7.3 - Implementing "The Gray Spot" strategies: A roadmap to personal evolution

- "The Power of Now: A Guide to Spiritual Enlightenment," Eckhart Tolle, New World Library, 1997 - Tolle explores the transformative power of present-moment awareness, guiding readers toward spiritual awakening and inner peace.
- "The Gifts of Imperfection: Let Go of Who You Think You're Supposed to Be and Embrace Who You Are," Brené Brown,

Hazelden Publishing, 2010 - Brown encourages embracing vulnerability and authenticity as pathways to wholehearted living and self-acceptance.

- "The Four Agreements: A Practical Guide to Personal Freedom," Don Miguel Ruiz, Amber-Allen Publishing, 1997 - Ruiz presents four principles for personal transformation, rooted in ancient Toltec wisdom and aimed at achieving inner peace and freedom.

10 Appendices

We can cite several examples of how a nation's specific policies and cultural values contribute to their residents' overall happiness around the world.

Nordic countries prioritize social support and social warfare programs, education, and work-life balance:
- Finland – "Sisu" – Encouraging resilience, determination, and courage in the face of adversity, finding purpose through strength of character.
- Denmark – "Hygge" – Creating a cozy and comfortable atmosphere, fostering well-being through simple pleasures and connections.
- Sweden – "Lagom" – Embracing balance and moderation for a life that is neither too much nor too little, promoting contentment and harmony.
- Norway – "Friluftsliv" – A strong connection to nature, seeking fulfillment through outdoor activities and appreciation of the natural world.

In the rest of *Europe*, depending on the local cultures and ways of living, similar concepts are observed:
- Switzerland – A high happiness ranking is linked to factors like a high standard of living, economic stability, quality healthcare, and a strong sense of community.
- Italy – "Dolce Far Niente" – Enjoying the sweetness of doing nothing, finding joy in leisure and relaxation.

- Netherlands – "Gezelligheid" – Embracing coziness and togetherness, finding warmth in shared moments with friends and loved ones.
- Ireland – "Sláinte" – Pursuing holistic well-being, including good health, happiness, and a positive, fulfilling life.
- Greece – "Meraki" – Infusing passion, love, and soul into everything one does, finding purpose through deep connection and dedication.

Similar cultural concepts related to leading a purposeful life are also widespread throughout the whole world, for example, the following ones.

In Asia
- Japan – "Ikigai" – Finding purpose at the intersection of what one loves, what one is good at, what the world needs, and what one can be paid for
- India – "Dharma" – Fulfilling moral and social obligations, following one's righteous path or duty.
- China – "Tao" – Aligning with the natural order of things, emphasizing simplicity, humility, and harmony with the universe.
- Thailand – "Sanuk" – Embracing pleasure and joy in all activities, promoting a lighthearted and fun approach to life.
- Russia – "Dusha" – Nurturing the Russian soul through art, literature, and deep connections with others.
- Iran – "Faravahar" – Representing the eternal soul and the path of righteousness, guiding individuals towards a purposeful and virtuous life.
- Bhutan - Gross National Happiness (GNH) – Measuring progress with a focus on sustainable development, environmental conservation, cultural preservation, and mental well-being.

In Africa
- Ghana – "Sankofa" – Learning from the past to move forward, embracing history and experiences for a purposeful life.

- South Africa – "Ubuntu" – Emphasizing interconnectedness and shared humanity, finding purpose through relationships with others and the community.
- Kenya – "Harambee" – Fostering collective effort and community collaboration, to achieve common goals, finding purpose through unity.

In America
- Mexico – "Comunidad" – Emphasizing community and strong social ties, mutual support, and collective well-being.
- Brazil – "Saudade" – Expressing a deep, melancholic longing for something or someone, emphasizing the beauty in bittersweet aspects of life.
- Hawaii – "Pono" – Seeking righteousness, balance, and harmony in all aspects of life for a sense of well-being.